Congratulations on your decision to buy this book. Working with Joe Klemczewski and Kori Propst, I transformed from burned-out corporate executive to Australia's most decorated fitness model. I cannot recommend them highly enough. I am excited for you—big things are ahead!

—JACQUII ALEXANDER, MBA, Ms. Bikini America, Model
Universe Champion, Physiotherapist & Businesswoman

In my business, eating well and finding time to work out often take a backseat to catching the next plane or staying out late for that big post-game interview. Joe and Kori's book was just what I needed to get on track and stay there.

—JOSH PAHIGIAN, MFA, Author of popular baseball travel books like
The Ultimate Baseball Road Trip and 101 Baseball Places to See Before You
Strike Out. His articles about sports travel have also appeared
on ESPN.com and in Men's Health.

Dr. Joe and Kori provide the keys to wellness and an enjoyable healthy lifestyle that's easy to understand for everyone. You don't even need to be a brain surgeon to figure it out.

—GREGORY J. LOOMIS, MD, PhD, Neurosurgeon

During my tenure as Editorial Director at Chelo Publishing, Joe and Kori were my two most popular contributors to our fitness magazines. Their combined understanding of exercise, sports psychology, and nutrition is unparalleled.

—RICH FITTER, Founder of the Drug-Free Athletes Coalition

If you are looking to rediscover what it feels like to have energy, a positive outlook, great health and an athletic physique, then this is the book for you. Dr. Joe and Kori are a unique team combining the best insights and learnings from nutritional science, physique development, and mental frameworks to achieve your goals. As a busy executive with constant international travel, Joe and Kori helped me transform my health, physique, and mental toughness to my best ever.

—DONAL BYRNE, CEO Corvil Inc.

The
Diet Doc

50 DAYS TO
Your Best
Body Life!

Joe Klemczewski, PhD
Kori Propst, PhD(c), LCMHC, LPC

The Diet Doc, LLC
8601 N. Kentucky Ave., Suite G
Evansville, IN 47725
(812) 868-8710, ext. 224
dr.joe@thedietdoc.com

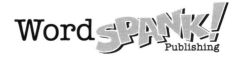

TABLE OF CONTENTS

ON THE SURFACE, the reason for obesity seems straightforward: people eat more in energy than they spend in physical activity; the excess is stored as fat and the weight goes up. The solution appears simple as well: exercise some willpower, push away from the table, and move more. But a deeper look quickly reveals that obesity has become one of the most complex and vexing global problems of modern life. Fifty years ago, obesity was scarce, only being a problem in a few developed countries such as the United States, England, and Australia. In 1970, less than 15 percent of American adults and less than 5 percent of children aged 6 to 19 years were obese. Currently, according to the CDC's 2012 survey of American health, 69 percent of adults and 33 percent of children aged 6 to 19 years are overweight or obese; 31 percent of those adults' and 17 percent of those childrens' weights meet the obesity criteria. Collectively, Americans carry more than four and a half billion excess pounds, an average of 14 pounds per person.

The obesity problem affects our already-strained healthcare system, our national productivity and security, and our quality of life. The CDC estimates that obesity is associated with 112,000 deaths per year and has been implicated in increased risk of atherosclerosis, hypertension, diabetes, heart and vascular disease, fatty liver and gall bladder disease, some types of cancer, dementia, sleep apnea, and arthritis. The medical care costs of obesity in the United States are staggering, totaling approximately $147 billion annually. Additionally, economists at Duke University found that obesity costs America more than $73 billion each year in lost productivity (lost earning potential). Regarding national security, between 1995 and 2008 the military rejected more than 140,000 recruits due to not meeting weight standards. Today, it's estimated that one in four young Americans do not meet the weight requirements to join the Armed Forces. There is also a stunning social penalty for being overweight. Overweight people are treated differently from their normal weight peers in educational, medical, and employment settings, even when their qualifications are the same.

In the U.S., we spend more than $40 billion each year on diet products and services trying not to be fat: that's more than the GDP of half of the world's nations. We *really* don't want to be fat. As much as we wish there was one thing in the fight against fat we could point to and change, there isn't. Whether you look at individuals or at society as a whole, the cause is complex. A combination of factors has eroded the ability of vast numbers of people to make healthy choices. As individuals, it's the sum total of our hundreds of little daily decisions regarding food and physical activity that results in us eating a little too much and moving too little; over time, that adds up to a lot of pounds. For the nation, our obesity problem has been magnified by the actions of industry, agriculture, and government, shaping the environment in which we live, work, and play. Often unintentionally, this makes it harder for us to make healthy choices. Big decisions made by industry, agriculture, and government have a huge impact on what we reach for when we're hungry and how long we sit at our desks and in our cars. For example, much of our food is consumed (and thus choices made) in schools, workplaces, and public settings. Similarly, how often we select walking as a mode of transportation, or how physically active we may be, are influenced by the availability of sidewalks and recreational areas within our community.

On an individual level, the journey to a healthier body, and healthier life, is paved by the thousands of behavioral decisions we make everyday regarding food choice and physical activity. In *50 Days*, Joe and Kori position you with key resources to optimize those decisions, thus resulting in attainable and sustainable weight loss. For decades, The Diet Doc team has guided thousands of clients, from housewives, to professional athletes, to physique competitors whittling that last one percent body fat, achieve and maintain their specific goals. Dr. Joe confers an understanding of nutrition and metabolism in an entertaining (and *almost* painless) fashion. More importantly, he demonstrates how to use that knowledge strategically (with respect to macronutrient content, quality, and timing) to maximize the body's "fat-incinerating" potential while simultaneously incorporating flexibility for compliance.

Research has shown that although exercise alone is not an effective weight-loss strategy, it is crucial in weight maintenance. Dr. Joe and Kori have created a challenging program that combines traditional resistance training, cardiovascular conditioning, and a functional training format that allow entry at virtually any skill level. With the Mental Edge, Kori Propst steers you internally to develop the mental, emotional, and behavioral skills necessary for permanent results.

A couple of final notes: 1. This is a journey best shared, rather than navigated solo; an on-going and reliable support system is crucial to success. Whether it's a formal group, family, friends from work or the gym, or an Internet chat room, the more like-minded people you have cheering you on, the better; 2. Planning ahead ensures default food choices are good quality and, with a little creativity, the workout gets accomplished. When I embarked on my personal journey, I was the single mother of teenage triplets; my workouts were often performed in 10- to 15-minute increments between shuttling my sons or daughter to various activities; 3. Detours are a certainty, embrace them as they take you in directions you thought not possible. As I progressed in weight training in my 40s, osteoarthritis of my right hip made itself known culminating in a hip replacement at age 46. It changed the way I approached exercise, but never stopped progress. At age 51 I achieved professional status in natural bodybuilding and last weekend (age 53) competed in my first powerlifting meet, benching, squatting, and deadlifting a combined total of 600.8 pounds. The greater the variety of healthy foods and physical activity with which you experiment, the spicier and more flavorful your life will be; 4. Embrace the changes in your lifestyle and celebrate those ever higher quality choices you make. Acting with intent confers great confidence and a sense of self-efficacy; 5. Never question the shadow you cast to influence those closest to you. My now 25-year-old children have adopted health behaviors from me that have put them miles ahead of where I was at their age.

The road rises open before you...enjoy the ride!

—Robin S. Berner, MD, MPH, MS, FACOEM

INTRODUCTION

FEW DAYS PASS in The Diet Doc office without somebody making a definitive statement about their metabolism.

"I don't eat much at all; my metabolism is a wreck."

"Once I turned thirty, my metabolism went downhill."

"Ever since *that* diet, my metabolism has never been the same."

"My problem is that I don't eat enough; I know that destroys your metabolism!"

I recently spoke with a young lady who had been gaining weight since puberty. In one stream of consciousness, she rambled through every reason she couldn't succeed. She told me she barely ate anything—sometimes just one meal per day. Nothing worked—she tried it all. My help wouldn't work, another diet wouldn't work, and she needed something easy—like a pill. As a matter of fact, by taking an over-the-counter "fat burner" she did lose forty-five pounds one year earlier.

I questioned her. "I thought nothing worked, but you say you lost forty-five pounds?" She attributed her success to that pill but couldn't answer why. "You said your metabolism was in such disrepair, you couldn't lose anything. A pill like that does very little to raise your metabolism, even acutely. It's likely that all it did was suppress your appetite so you ate less." She agreed that it had indeed curbed her appetite and she ate less.

"But you said your problem was that you didn't eat enough and you barely ate anything—if this pill made you eat less and you lost forty-five pounds, how did that work? And you said eating less lowers your metabolism. If your met rate dropped even further than the already-low level,

how did you lose?"

Blank stare.

Her mother chimed in to defend her, "She eats hardly anything—you should see her. Hardly anything!"

"Really? You're with her twenty-four hours a day? You watch everything she eats?" More questioning led the young lady to admit she was drinking enough Mountain Dew alone to put her in a calorie surplus—a two-liter most days. She also ate most meals in the restaurant where she worked, and she drank a lot of alcohol.

Not quite "nothing."

Is this the case with everyone struggling to lose weight? Are we a bunch of self-deceived victims of ignorance? Are we liars who closet-eat and binge? Or, do we have a national—even global—epidemic of mysterious metabolic suppression making us all fat?

Most people don't know how nutrition works inside (physiologically) or outside (behaviorally) the body any more than I know how the transmission in my Jeep works. We need to address both. Physiology and behavior—not my Jeep. You can eat in a way that increases your metabolism, there's no doubt about it. But, while we help you engage in the process of incinerating body fat, we want you to learn how and why it's happening so you don't get blindsided and knocked off track now or later.

This book will explain how your metabolism works, how to make sure it's functioning maximally, and will provide you with an exact plan to ramp you toward success. Just like the young lady who lost forty-five pounds only to gain it back, you have to be wary about regaining weight. Most of us have lost weight only to gain it back—and then some. Studies show that almost ninety-eight percent of people who lose weight regain it within two years. We have to start with the end in mind. It's not the "plan" you find in these pages that will keep you lean. The knowledge you gain and your own experience will be the bridge to a new body—maybe a new life!

Long-term success is the goal.

When we bought e-readers for our kids, the quick-start guide was a single page with six steps. The manual was over sixty pages. We consider this book a thorough treatise, but let's be honest, we all look for the "on" button before we ever open a user's manual. Check out our Rapid-Results Guide—we know you can't resist. We're actually thrilled to bring something so precise and innovative to you!

Most people don't understand how nutrition works inside (physiologically) or outside (behaviorally) the body any more than I know how the transmission in my Jeep works. We need to address both.

But don't be satisfied with just being able to lose weight—make this your last diet.

Here's a look at what's in store as you journey through this experience:

⚡ **SECTION 1 · Rapid Results Guide:** In just ten steps, you will be up and running toward permanent weight loss and an athletic life.

🜁 **SECTION 2 · Nutrition:** Learn how to build your metabolism to maximal levels by using precise meal planning, all made easy with a detailed exchange list.

💡 **SECTION 3 · Mental Edge:** No one can argue that the power of the mind is our greatest asset. Now you have all the tools you'll ever need for success!

⏱ **SECTION 4 · Metabolic Transformation Scholar**

🚫 **SECTION 5 · Recipes:** A companion to the meal exchange list, the recipe section provides categorized, tasty options that make eating enjoyable.

✗ **SECTION 6 · Training:** The Metabolic Inferno Fat-Incinerating Training System may be the most unique format ever created. Combining cutting-edge functional training with traditional strength and cardiovascular work, the progression possibilities are endless.

📄 **SECTION 7 · Appendix:** Don't skip these activities and resources—they meld the information into practice, help cultivate habits, and create permanence.

Take advantage of the Rapid Results Guide and dig in, but keep reading. You'll learn how your body stores and loses fat, and how to stay in a fat-loss-friendly eating pattern. You'll understand how you can have more energy, feel better, and keep nutrition easy with a powerful mindset. *50 Days* will throw you on the fast track and you'll be achieving goals before you know it. Think rocket fuel for your metabolism.

Let's start the fire!

SECTION 1:
Rapid Results Guide

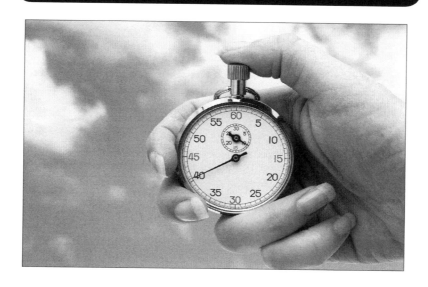

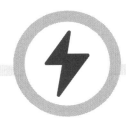

PARTS INCLUDED:

50 Days to Your Best ~~Body~~ *Life!* book.

- Permanent weight-loss schematic.

- Specific meal-planning instructions.

- Metabolic Inferno Fat-incinerating workout plan.

- Life-changing mindset tactics.

PARTS NOT INCLUDED:

✓ Your will to succeed—don't begin assembly without it.

✓ Advanced workout gear—not required, but recommended for progression:

- Stability ball (note size-per-height).

- Medicine ball (note weight per strength level).

- Small dumbbells (note weight per strength level).

- Exercise bands/tubing (note varying resistance levels).

- Exercise mat (note varying length and thicknesses).

- Stop watch or timer (simple is better).

- Headbands (Yes, they're back, and, yes, you will sweat!).

- Legwarmers (Kidding. The '80s are over...but headbands are back!).

STEPS:

Step 1: Read entire Rapid Results Guide.

Step 2: Map out your daily schedule, including meal times.

Step 3: Select a meal from each category and create a sample day (Refer to Chapters 4 through 9).

Step 4: Prepare necessary food.

Step 5: Plan ahead for meal variety and flexibility.

Step 6: Secure any necessary training aids.

Step 7: Consult physician for permission to proceed.

Step 8: Read the Fast Facts summary.

Step 9: Read the entire book, one chapter at a time, but start the program today.

Step 10: What are you waiting for? GO!

NUTRITION FAST FACTS:

Chapter One—Metabolism

- We all have different genetic metabolic rates.
- We can increase our metabolic rates functionally, up to our genetic maximum, with the right amount, right sources, and right combinations of food: targeted meals.
- Activity is the sledgehammer in moving metabolism upward.

Chapter Two—Thermogenesis

- Metabolism is affected by the digestion of different foods—the thermic effect of food.
- Each food source (protein, carbs, and fat)—and even different forms of each—require different levels of energy to digest.
- All three macronutrients play vital roles in health, energy, metabolism, and weight loss.

Chapter Three—Metabolic Positioning

- You can lose weight up to fifty percent faster—eating the same amount of calories—just by getting into the metabolic position to lose body fat and then staying there.
- Carbs are important for several reasons, but managing them properly allows faster fat burning.
- The right plan with a good measure of flexibility is the road map to effective metabolic positioning, but consistency is what keeps you there. Objectivity is king.

Chapter Four—Precision Meals

- Achieving sustainable and healthy fat loss requires a physiologically sound structure—no gimmicks.
- Rigid structure that doesn't account for real-life flexibility will fail every time.
- Different times of the day—different circumstances—are best met with a targeted, precise meal that allows for consistent fat loss, but provides energy, workout recovery, and hunger prevention.

TRAINING FAST FACTS:

Cardiovascular Components

- Progress at your own pace. Be safe.
- Maximum heart rate is 220 minus your age. Heart rate monitors are available at sporting goods stores, but you can also take your pulse for six seconds and multiply by ten to figure beats per minute.
- Take note of warm-up and stretching instructions. If you ever feel a muscle strain, discontinue exercise and only continue at pain-free intensity levels and with exercises that are pain free. Consult a health care professional if necessary.

Strength Training Components

- Varying weight or resistance levels of exercise bands, dumbbells, and medicine balls can help with progress, but you can begin without any equipment.
- Each week progresses in movement difficulty, time, or intensity, but you can also progress within the beginner, intermediate, and advanced levels.
- Traditional gym equipment can be used to replicate many movements with much greater resistance. With some open space, this program can be performed in a commercial training facility.

Functional Training Components

- Though many functional movements don't require any equipment, they can still be quite challenging. Make sure your shoulders, knees, and back are safe and pain free.
- Form is critical for functional exercises—master execution before advancing.
- Effort is the driving force of progress. Full range of motion, maximal exertion, and pace are yours to control. Even the beginner-level exercises can challenge an experienced athlete if work output is great enough.

MENTAL EDGE FAST FACTS:

Chapter Ten—Eliminating Barriers

- Permanent weight loss requires a focus on the psychology of eating behavior.
- Poor adherence to diets is often a result of severe restriction, rigid rules, lack of flexibility, and poor emotional management skills.
- Dieters show a greater tendency to overeat during times of emotional stress and compensate for perceived dieting failures by eating more.
- Emotional eating is a symptom of thinking and feeling errors.

Chapter Eleven—Utilizing Our Internal Voices

- Change requires acting with intention and avoiding impulsive behavior. Pause, think, and determine the most optimal course of action that is in line with your goals.
- Take responsibility and identify your choices rather than assuming there is only one option.
- Notice what you pay attention to and how you perceive your circumstances.
- Individuals who keep their weight off permanently do not adopt a "quick-fix" approach and they learn how to delay gratification.
- Emotional intelligence skills increase your mind and body awareness so you can respond with less judgment and more control.
- Emotional and binge eating is not about food. Learning how to be comfortable with discomfort decreases your reliance on food to cope with emotion.

Chapter Twelve—Moving from Motivation to Commitment

- Motivation is influenced by mood, is situational, and will wax and wane depending on your circumstances.
- Commitment is an *I will do whatever it takes* attitude.
- Moving from being motivated to being committed requires perspective-taking and reminding yourself of the reasons for wanting to change, so that when challenges arise, you will keep on trucking.

Chapter Thirteen—Taking Risks: Developing a Growth Mindset

- Our basic need for safety/avoiding harm often blocks our willingness to step out of our comfort zones.
- Practicing a growth mindset enables movement toward challenges and greater persistence in the face of setbacks.

- Establishing your "why" will help transition your goal from extrinsic to intrinsic.
- Asking yourself tough questions will help you learn about your personal roadblocks.

Chapter Fourteen—Environmental Triggers

- Eating is triggered by internal and external mechanisms.
- We make over 200 food-related decisions on a daily basis.
- Overweight and obese individuals are more responsive to environmental food cues and perceive greater rewards attached to food.
- Your motivation to eat is influenced by the associations and meanings you have attached to food, as well as the environment.
- To change your eating habits, you must train your brain through repeatedly thinking and behaving differently.

Chapter Fifteen—Maintenance: Be a Life Athlete!

- Maintaining a permanently lean and healthy body, and a strong, positive mindset, requires attention.
- All-or-nothing thinking errors, or making assumptions, leaves us vulnerable to actions that are often outside of our best interests.
- Flexibility (in thought and action) is a key component of permanent weight loss.
- Problem-solving is action oriented and involves recognition, acknowledgement, defining, assessment, reflection, and responding.
- Successful weight loss maintenance involves proactively managing emotion and flexibility with food intake and exercise.
- Threats to your goal can have a positive impact on the effort you exert toward meeting it. Asking yourself "what might go wrong?" gives you the ability to plan ahead for damage mitigation.
- Individuals who meet their goals think with a growth-oriented mindset. They value challenge and use setbacks to improve their strategy for success.
- Exercise is a key component of successful weight maintenance and overall health.
- Those who regain their weight report the effort it takes to maintain as being almost impossible. The longer maintenance is reported, however, the more automatic the required behaviors become.
- Support is a crucial component for weight-loss success and long-term maintenance.

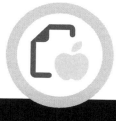

SECTION 2:
Nutrition

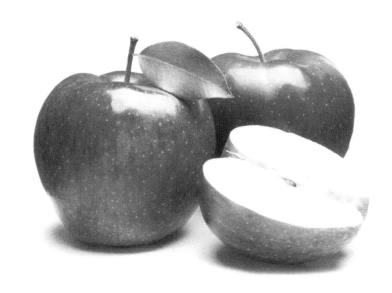

CHAPTER ONE

Metabolism

MORE MISINFORMATION REGARDING metabolism is pouring into the internet than ever before. Bloggers are scaring people into thinking their metabolism is being wrecked permanently, pseudo-experts claim to have the cure, marketers are hawking the latest miracle, and the consumer is left to wonder what they should have for dinner. Let's cover some basics.

Metabolism: the chemical process by which cells produce the substances and energy needed to sustain life. As part of metabolism, organic compounds are broken down to provide heat and energy in the process called catabolism. Simpler molecules are also used to build more complex compounds like proteins for growth and repair of tissues as part of anabolism. Many metabolic processes are brought about by the action of enzymes. The overall speed at which an organism carries out its metabolic processes is termed its metabolic rate (or, when the organism is at rest, its basal metabolic rate). Birds, for example, have a high metabolic rate, since they are warm-blooded, and their usual method of locomotion, flight, requires large amounts of energy. Accordingly, birds usually need large amounts of high-quality, energy-rich foods such as seeds or meat, which they must eat frequently. See more at "cellular respiration." (*The American Heritage Science Dictionary*. Houghton Mifflin Company. 2005.)

Now you remember why you didn't want to grow up to be a molecular biologist. Or maybe you're checking Amazon's return policy for bad books. I promise the rest of *50 Days* won't put you to sleep, but there is some rich information packed into that definition that we need to pick apart. You're going to learn how to control your metabolism!

Cellular

Chemical process…cells…substances…energy… blah, blah, blah. Think of it this way: your metabolism isn't just a magic dial spinning like the electrical meter on the back of your house. There is a reason we need food—the cells of our body need it to work, grow, repair, and do cell things. Red blood cells do red blood cell things,

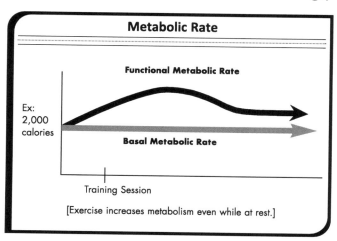

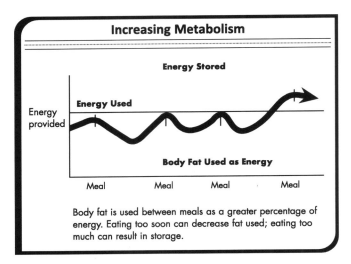

Increasing Metabolism

Energy Stored

Energy Used

Energy provided

Body Fat Used as Energy

Meal   Meal   Meal   Meal

Body fat is used between meals as a greater percentage of energy. Eating too soon can decrease fat used; eating too much can result in storage.

kidney cells do kidney cell things, and brain cells sit around on Sunday and watch ESPN—it's pure biology.

The core of how much energy we need—how much food we have to consume—is in the hands of every little cell in our bodies. Trillions of little cells. The cell is the most basic unit of life. They're often described as little factories, or even cities. Cells have transportation systems, waste removal systems, energy production facilities, and the list goes on. Basal metabolic rate goes hand in hand with the needs of the cell. Whether you're on a treadmill or asleep, a brain cell has to stay alive, process nutrients, and keep the show rolling. The same goes for a nerve cell, a skin cell, and a big toe cell. Okay, I made that one up; there's no such thing as a big toe cell.

Basal metabolic rate is an average energy measurement at rest. We all know that when we start exercising, we

> I know you've been taught carbs are evil little creatures, but they play a very important role in helping you lose body fat!

burn more calories. Our heart is beating faster, our muscles are working harder, and—refer back to the mention of heat in the definition above—we sweat. Since our muscular system is working harder, thus driving the greater demand for energy (calories), every cell in our body also gets a boost in activity. More oxygen is carried to cells via increased blood flow, nutrients are carried around faster, waste is carried away sooner—the body is in motion down to the smallest unit of life! This makes exercise a dominant way of increasing metabolism immediately—what I call functional metabolism. The metabolism will even stay elevated for some time after the activity has stopped. Moderate exercise may result in an extra hour of enhanced calorie burning, but intense training can extend that time up to several hours. One recent study concluded that the body benefits from an enhanced ability to burn fatty acids as energy for a full day after exercise. Metabolism involves every cell and we can affect it by how and what we eat, as well as with exercise.

Increasing activity obviously makes us warmer, but here's something that may be new to you: eating increases metabolism as well. My son's baseball team had an all-you-can-eat pancake breakfast fundraiser on a Saturday morning. Several of the team moms thought it was a riot to see me serving pancakes wearing a Diet Doc baseball cap, but, hey; we were on a mission to get these boys to the Little League World Series! My wife commented later, "Wow, did they put something in those pancakes? After three of them I started sweating—I was so hot!" Naturally, I offered that it might have just been seeing me in an apron that got her all revved up. In reality, it's a good reminder of what carbs do. They're very thermogenic—they create a spike in metabolism as the body quickly shuttles the digested glucose around to be used...or stored if you eat too much. I know you've been taught carbs are evil little creatures, but they play a very important role in helping you *lose* body fat!

Heat and Energy

The words anabolism and catabolism used in the definition of metabolism refer to the building or breaking down of material within the body. If the body has an influx of nutrients, cells have what they need to repair and build. This activity creates a heat transfer—a literal production of heat. Have you ever eaten so much food at one time that you start sweating, just as my wife did after eating pancakes? How about eating so much that you can feel and hear your heart beating significantly harder than normal? Come on, fess up; I know you have! That is the effect of thermogenesis and the thermic potential of food. Thermogenesis and thermic effect are concepts we're going to build on through the next chapter. It's where the metabolic money is at.

It takes energy to digest, assimilate, transport, and utilize—metabolize—the food we eat. This is one reason for the mantra "eat smaller, more frequent meals." The more frequently we eat, the more instances we nudge our metabolism higher. Obviously there is a law of diminishing returns. If we eat too much per meal, we store body fat. If we eat too often, we don't give ourselves the time between meals to tap into body fat stores for energy. Both are major factors in weight loss and potential plateaus—I'd underline them if I were you. Go ahead and get your highlighter. Start with "If we eat too much..." and end with "...body fat stores for energy." How much you eat, how you divide that food into meals, and how much comes from protein, carbohydrates, and fat, are all variables that create the foundation of your success.

Birds?

Dictionaries have become more descriptive since my grade-school days. The example of a bird with a fast-beating heart, a swift rate of locomotion, and a constant need for energy, provides a fantastic look at metabolism! Compare the bird to a slow-moving elephant. Sure, the elephant needs substantially more food due to its size, but pound for pound, the bird needs more. I'll pause for a second to let that sink in. It's true—a bird needs more food than an elephant.

A great white shark spends its entire day looking for food. A mature great white can weigh 5,000 pounds and eat 500 pounds of food every day. As impressive as that sounds, it's only ten percent of its body weight while a bat will eat thirty percent of its weight in mosquitos in one night. Crazy, I know. You can cancel your subscription to *National Geographic*; all you need is *The Diet Doc*. In addition to the fun animal facts you can use to impress your office mates, keep one point in mind: activity increases metabolism.

> If we eat too much per meal, we store body fat. If we eat too often, we don't give ourselves the time between meals to tap into body fat stores for energy.

DNA

The strict definition of metabolism leaves out the most important part to us individually. In a world of advertising pitchmen screaming how their pill, potion, or program can give you the body of a model in two weeks, not many people like to talk about the fact that metabolism is largely genetically determined. We all know someone who eats a tremendous amount of food and stays lean. Others may be heavy as a child and remain a larger person through life. As parents, we optimistically call them big-boned, husky, stocky, and solid, but that can do little to blunt the issue.

There are many differences in the endocrine system, neural-gastric loop, and even the sheer number of body fat cells from one person to another. The fact that some people have a much harder time losing weight is not in dispute at all. I'm a bullhorn champion trying to explain the metabolic uniqueness person to person. However, the topic at hand is how much the metabolism can be improved from whatever baseline is normal for you. You can underperform metabolically, or you can accelerate cellular activity to maximal levels, by how you eat and through activity.

> You can underperform metabolically, or you can accelerate cellular activity to maximal levels, by how you eat and through activity.

Health Complications

A number of hormonal complications can bring a normal metabolism to its knees. Low thyroid function, menopausal changes, and many other health issues can legitimately be blamed. Though only typical in around five percent of the population, if you feel there are abnormal obstructions to your progress, it can be worth a trip to the doctor for some blood work to find out. I recently suggested to four clients that they might have hormonal issues underlying their slow loss pace. Every one of them tested at clinically low levels of thyroid hormone or testosterone. It's not common, but it does happen.

Obesity is prevalent in my family and it has always been obvious to me that my metabolism is on the slow end of the continuum. I've never used that as an excuse to keep from being healthy, but when comparing my food needs to an average male, I can't afford to be a super-size-me eater. When I turned forty I underwent my first hormonal panel and found I'm sub-clinically hypothyroid. As nice as it is to have confirmation that there's a reason for not being able to eat as much as others, it doesn't change a thing. It's relative. If someone else has a metabolism that requires 3,000 calories per day, and my body only uses 2,000 calories per day, I won't be any hungrier on a 500-calorie deficit (1,500 calories) than they would be (2,500 calories). Sure, they still get more slices of pizza (and I hate that!), but it's relative to our individual metabolic rates. If there is a medical problem, get the help you need. If you're on the lower end of normal, let's build to your genetic max. If you're one of the rare, freakishly-high metabolic monsters who can eat all day and never gain a pound, you probably don't need this book. Get a refund and buy a Big Mac.

CHAPTER TWO

Thermogenesis

NOW THAT YOU understand metabolism—I promise I won't put you through that again—let's keep digging. Your total energy expenditure includes your basal metabolic rate and what you use in above-normal activity. There's another part of the calorie balance sheet that you may not be aware of. Diet-induced thermogenesis can add five- to fifteen-percent more to the calorie outflow bottom line. Your resting metabolic rate makes up sixty- to seventy-percent of your energy output and activity adds thirty- to forty-percent.

Let me explain. When food is consumed, it requires energy to digest and assimilate the nutrients. Each macronutrient (protein, carbohydrate, and fat) has a different effect on metabolism based on its diet-induced rate of thermogenesis. Protein has the greatest thermic effect at twenty- to thirty-percent. It takes twenty- to thirty-percent of the calories consumed from a protein source to actually digest and assimilate it.

This is where some bloggers and freelance writers often fall short. When we eat, we burn more calories. *So, let's all eat more! If you're not losing weight, you're not eating enough!* That logic eerily sounds like our government trying to spend its way out of debt. Protein has the highest thermic effect at twenty- to thirty-percent. The other seventy- to eighty-percent of the calories have to be used...or stored. Just because it takes energy to digest food—temporarily increasing metabolism—we still have to *need* that food.

Recall that energy is a measurement of heat or heat loss. A high thermic effect of a food or meal shows a higher level of work is being done to digest that food. Fat has the lowest thermic potential at barely five percent. Carbs have a bit of a range, being measured at five- to thirty-percent. I contend there's more to the story with carbohydrates—a lot more. Actually, it's the reason behind the large range of measured thermic effect that makes it one of the greatest secrets to weight loss—especially

> A high thermic effect of a food or meal shows a higher level of work is being done to digest that food.

Thermic Effect of Food		
Protein	**20-30%**	*of calories used during digestion and assimilation*
Carbs	**5-30%**	*of calories used during digestion and assimilation*
Fat	**0-5%**	*of calories used during digestion and assimilation*

Protein and complex carbohydrates boost metabolism.

in the current anti-carb movement. Recall the image of my wife sweating while eating pancakes? Wait a minute, don't think about my wife sweating; stop that!

Protein

Let's sprint through a quick review of protein. Protein is made up of amino acids, the building blocks for cells and tissues. Amino acids are also used as the catalysts in biochemical reactions, essential for all bodily processes. Because the structure of protein is so complex, it takes more time and more energy to digest and assimilate, thus the higher thermic potential. From a dietary perspective, it has also been proven to have a significantly positive influence on fullness, or satiety. Slower digestion, higher thermic potential, less hunger, muscle-building potential—what's not to love about protein?

> "Getting enough protein in each day through critical meals—targeted meals—can increase thermogenesis, lead to greater health, lower hunger, and increase recovery from workouts."

Many answer that jest quite literally by constructing diets with more protein than the body can use, and this has two negative impact points. The first is that once your body has as much protein as it can utilize, more does not create increased anabolism (muscle-building). Too much can cause higher levels of acidosis, which can be stressful to your liver and kidneys. Debates rage whether or not large amounts of dietary protein cause damage, but it is not questioned that high levels cause increased liver enzyme levels, BUN (blood urea nitrogen) levels, and kidney stress. There is no upside, only risk. Getting enough protein each day through critical meals—targeted meals—can increase thermogenesis, lead to greater health, lower hunger, and increase recovery from workouts. The right amount is the right amount. Too much is potentially harmful and too little creates unwanted deficits.

Fat

The spotlight on fat intake changes as diet fads cycle in and out of vogue, but it's always in the mix. Contrast the no-fat plans to Atkins and other ketogenic diets. Our culture has virtually banned trans-fats—some cities have!—and is embracing essential fats with positive-spin articles in every health magazine. Most people will recognize fat source discussions regarding hormone production and brain health. Others now look for the individual health benefits of various oils and fats like olive oil, grape seed oil, flax seed oil, and now even saturated sources like coconut oil.

Recent attention has been given to the value of "natural" fats as long as they are organic and unadulterated. I know people who milk their own goats to consume unpasteurized, fresh, whole milk and eat a diet high in fat due to the over-reaching attention

> Don't lose sight of what we already know when looking at novel information: too much fat is stored as body fat regardless how good the source.

given to healthier versions of fat. Don't lose sight of what we already know when looking at novel information: too much fat is stored as body fat regardless how good the source. Essential fatty acids are...essential, but remember the thermic potential is the lowest of any macronutrient—zero-to five-percent. Essential fatty acids are important, but consistent intake can be measured weekly or monthly, it doesn't have to be daily.

Carbs

This is where it gets fun. The resurgence of low-carb/ketogenic diets has created a generation of people who assume carbs make you fat. Excess carbs will be stored as body fat—as will excessive amounts of any macronutrient. True. But, carbohydrates are the body's preferred source of energy; that makes them a double-edged sword. When carbs are present—blood sugar from a recently-eaten meal, stored carbs (glycogen) in the liver, or glycogen in the muscle—they can and will be used if there is an energy deficit. Carbohydrate naysayers would say that when carbs are taken out of the diet the body will use fat sooner and in higher percentages. Also true. Case closed, right? We should all stop eating carbs! Not exactly. This is where we need to apply a little *CSI: Diet Doc.*

When you eliminate carbs, you have the greatest potential to slash your metabolism. Studies show that a low-carb diet can decrease your metabolism by almost fifty percent in just a couple of months. While your body is catabolizing fat for energy, without carbs as a buffer, you also use more amino acids for energy—you lose lean body mass. Decreasing your metabolic rate and losing muscle—sound like a good diet plan to you? Carbs have a purpose. When protein levels are adequate, nothing increases metabolism and gives the potential for muscle gain like carbs. Even if gaining muscle is not your goal, maintaining it should be. Carbs are the most metabolic and anabolic macronutrient we consume once protein intake is sufficiently in place.

> When protein levels are adequate, nothing increases metabolism and gives the potential for muscle gain like carbs.

I keep saying "when protein is adequate" because protein contains the amino acids necessary for building and repairing cells. Protein intake has to be suitable per day—and preferably meal by meal—but once those levels have been met, more is not helpful. Many make the mistake of continuing to increase protein and to limit carbs, but, comparatively, that approach is inferior for stimulating metabolism and creating the potential for lean body mass gains. Carbs are needed.

The best way of understanding macronutrients is to ditch the view that one is better than another or that any of them is "bad." All three have necessary roles and all three can be harmful in excess. Using the right amount at the right time makes all the difference. Quality and source selection each play a role, but precise and targeted planning of your meals will give you a colossal advantage. We'll even show you how sugary foods can function as optimal choices in some contexts. Bring on the Reese's!

Energy and Thermogenesis

Thermic potential is a linear equation—it takes a specific amount of energy to digest and assimilate the nutritional constituents of the food we eat. However, recall the nuance that this can actually be a bit of a range. The complexity of each macronutrient can change its thermic potential. For example, difference sources of carbohydrates can be at opposite ends of the glycemic index continuum. Two other points to consider are 1) the combination of macronutrients in the meal, and 2) the sheer size of the meal. There are times of the day when you may want a meal with no carbohydrates, all carbohydrates, complex carbohydrates, or even simple carbs. This is perhaps the greatest example of how you can use the right macronutrients, in the right amount, and at the right time to achieve your best results.

Following chapters will outline why time of day and how unique circumstances can dictate what type of meal is best. There are instances where a protein-only meal is your best option, a small snack should be utilized, or your biggest meal of the day should be mowed down like an all-you-can-eat buffet at the mercy of an NFL lineman. This is a huge point: protein does have the highest consistent thermic potential, but carbs can weigh in with up to a thirty-percent thermic effect. It's important to target the right meals with the right macronutrients and ratios to fuel (heat loss) the best activity (functional metabolism). In other words, it's the merger of the thermic effect of food, the quantity of each, and activity that determines how efficiently the calories eaten will be used. Timing, timing, timing. Function, function, function. Less hunger, more energy, better results from training, higher overall met rate...booyah!

CHAPTER THREE

Metabolic Positioning

HAVE YOU EVER lost weight only to gain it back? Dumb question, I know. You may be thinking about the times you've lost twenty or thirty pounds only to watch the numbers on the scale creep up again. Maybe even a hundred pounds. I'm referring, though, to losing two or three pounds—maybe four or five— and just days later experiencing a quick regain. Some repeat this cycle week after week, only to feel they may never get lean. A client recently exclaimed just as much. After riding that same weekly yo-yo for a couple of months, she cried, "I'm a freak of nature!"

She started losing at a good clip: ten pounds in ten weeks. With confirmed hormonal insufficiencies, that's a super pace! Then a little binge occurred and she had to lose a couple of the same pounds again.

Then again.

And again.

Two and a half months of perfect, steady progress was followed by two and a half months of standing still. Is she a freak of nature or is her inconsistency slowing her down?

Another client who had a very fast metabolism and lost weight quickly also ran into a plateau. Week after week I racked my brain and made changes to her plan, looking for a way to ramp her

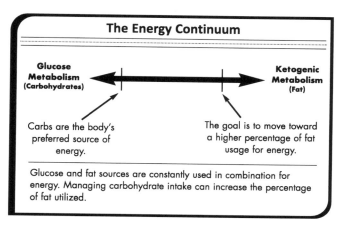

The Energy Continuum

Glucose Metabolism (Carbohydrates) ← → Ketogenic Metabolism (Fat)

Carbs are the body's preferred source of energy.

The goal is to move toward a higher percentage of fat usage for energy.

Glucose and fat sources are constantly used in combination for energy. Managing carbohydrate intake can increase the percentage of fat utilized.

metabolism back to a higher level. After months of frustration—for both of us—she admitted, "Oh, yeah, I was binging like a fiend the whole time and lying to you." Is she a freak of nature too?

Yet another client was losing so painfully slow that I spent weeks trying to hunt down the perfect combination of foods, meals, and macrontrient levels. I would have been happy to see her weight-loss pace just begin to crawl! One day she offered, "I didn't know Tic-Tacs had calories—I've been eating five boxes a day. Five boxes! That's over a hundred grams of sugar (carbohydrate) per day that was unaccounted for!

Freak of nature?

I recall a young man who came in for an initial consultation. He was so excited to get started that he purchased my book and began dieting a week

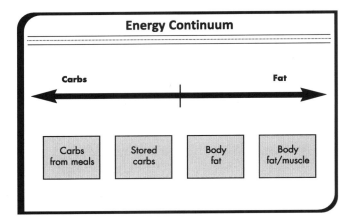

prior. He said, "I lost ten pounds in the first week!" I began to explain how he had already put himself in a metabolic position where he was now losing body fat maximally, but he cut me off. "Knowing I was coming to see you Monday, my friends and I went out Saturday and ate pizza and drank beer—a lot of it. I gained eleven pounds; I'm starting over."

Sound familiar?

There's a reason that losing weight is more than counting calories. Did you know that you can eat the same amount of calories and lose up to fifty percent more body fat in the same amount of time? What you eat, the quality of foods you eat, the combination of foods, meal timing, and a host of other variables will affect your speed of loss, but there is a greater factor at play. There's something I like to call metabolic positioning.

The Carb Buffer Zone

"I lost seven pounds this week, but I know it was all water." We so quickly discount that first drop on the scale as if it's not important. I'm sure it's because the loss is often so fleeting—as with my pizza-and-beer client. But, if that first step was understood as a portal to a new world of fast fat loss, we might be a little more excited about it.

It is not only the door to faster fat loss, but

consistent progress.

Consistent.

Your body can use any macronutrient as energy, and we have stored versions of those same sources. Every cell in your body—over sixty trillion at last estimate—needs second-by-second glucose: blood sugar. The fastest way to get glucose to those cells comes from breaking down a carbohydrate source. When we eat carbohydrates, we're giving our body what our cells need. That's a double-edged sword because we want our body to use the body fat we're trying to lose. We have to limit our carb intake to force our bodies to use stored fat, but we house a few hundred grams of carbs in our body that we have to work through before that will happen.

Your body will use carbs first for energy, not body fat. That means carbs must be reduced below the normal level that would satisfy energy requirements. But, if you drop them too low, metabolic rate can gradually—or rapidly depending on your approach—be suppressed to the point that it's almost impossible to lose weight. You must keep carbs high enough to prevent this, but a large enough reduction has to be employed so that your body seeks an alternative source of energy: body fat. This is quite a balancing act!

The carb buffer zone is what your body

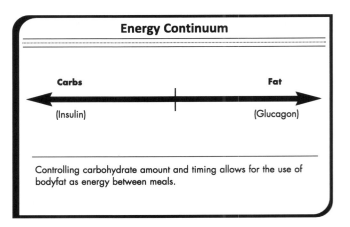

Controlling carbohydrate amount and timing allows for the use of bodyfat as energy between meals.

> We have to limit our carb intake to force our bodies to use stored fat, but we house a few hundred grams of carbs in our body that we have to work through before that will happen.

maintains internally as glycogen: the stored form of glucose. We stash some in our liver and a bunch in our muscle. If you reduce carbs moderately, you can safely deplete glycogen stores in your body to the point body fat is used maximally within two to four days. That's where you want to be. Your metabolism is safe, but you're losing body fat consistently. If you push too fast, your metabolism will suffer and progress can come to a halt.

On a side note, stored carbs hold water like a sponge. When you start using this stored glycogen, you release that water, and water is heavy—almost nine pounds per gallon. Indeed, a lot of the initial weight lost on a diet is water, but it's because you are working through stored carbs, which puts you in a *position to lose body fat*.

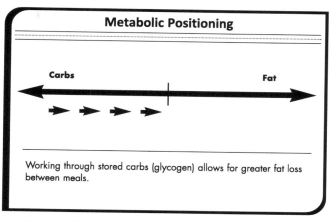

Metabolic Positioning

Carbs   Fat

Working through stored carbs (glycogen) allows for greater fat loss between meals.

Metabolic positioning.

That is huge!

Working through those internal carbs takes days, but it's the only way you start using body fat as energy consistently. Even before you throttle your body with advanced techniques and knowledge regarding thermogenesis, you have to know how to get to and stay in this metabolic position.

Living on the Edge

Your goal is to lose as fast as you can—I know—but it is imperative that it's not a short-term loss that sets you up for massive regain. I hereby charge you with the epic mission of pushing your metabolism higher *while* keeping one eye on the long-term successful transition to easy, stress-free maintenance. It's a big deal. Getting yourself to that perfect balance point may seem like living on the edge of a razor, but it doesn't have to be difficult. Let us do the heavy lifting and your job is simply to take your time, learn, and implement well. We want this to be your last diet ever!

The plan we have mapped out moves you through this moderate glycogen depletion and into consistent fat loss. That is the first step—it pushes you through the doorway to real fat loss. You'll also experience increasing energy for workouts

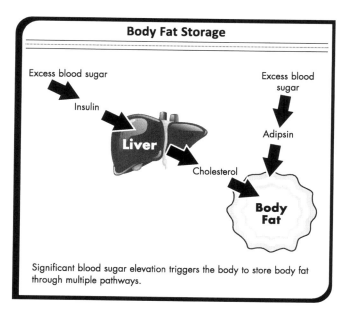

Body Fat Storage

Excess blood sugar

Insulin

Liver

Excess blood sugar

Adipsin

Cholesterol

Body Fat

Significant blood sugar elevation triggers the body to store body fat through multiple pathways.

so you can reshape and build your best physique, recover well from training, feel better, stay as metabolically powerful as possible, and start living an enthusiastic life. Any objections to that?

But Dr. Atkins said...

Too much carbohydrate in one meal will cause body fat gain right now and too much carb in a day or a week will keep the fat train rolling. All of the early ketogenic (low-carb) proponents were right to focus on carbs; they just took it too far. Your body can use a limited amount of carbohydrate at a time and when more is eaten, a torrent of storage processes occurs. As carbohydrate is digested into glucose (blood sugar), it's packed into the liver and muscle to be stored. At the same time, the liver starts converting some into cholesterol to be stored as fat and fat cells start pulling glucose in to be converted to body fat directly. That's a lot of storing!

When you consume more carbohydrate than you can use right then, body fat is the result—think Pac-Man on meth.

How much is too much? That's the question everyone wishes they could answer with a magic eight ball. (Do they still make those?) It depends on your metabolism, how much and when you last ate—even what your food intake has been for days prior, and what your preceding activity level has been. It could range from twenty grams of carbs to forty or fifty grams typically. Do a little math on a "normal" meal in society and it may be apparent why two-thirds of us are overweight. On that note, did you know researchers predict around *half* of Americans will be obese by 2030? Not you, my fat-burning friend; not you. You are becoming a metabolic inferno!

The Rest of the Story

Carbs get the twenty-million-dollar lead role, but protein and fat round out a complete cast. Many would interpret the fact that too much carb intake can easily lead to fat gain and throw the baby out with the bath water. Why not just eliminate carbs? Carbs are the most metabolically potent macronutrient we eat. If you drop them too low, within a couple of months your metabolism is plummeting. They're also very anabolic—important to gain or maintain lean body mass and overall health. If you're consuming enough protein to meet dietary needs, more won't create additional muscle-building benefit...but more carbohydrate will. Again I repeat: we need to manage carbs to avoid gaining weight. We need to reduce them to lose weight, but carbs are critically important—we can't drop them completely.

Low-carb diets ask you to increase your protein and/or fat to high levels, or simply make them "free"—eat all you want. One premise is due to the high thermic potential of protein. If it takes almost a third of the calories eaten from protein just to digest it, why not keep eating? It's like getting thirty percent off of your favorite sneakers—why

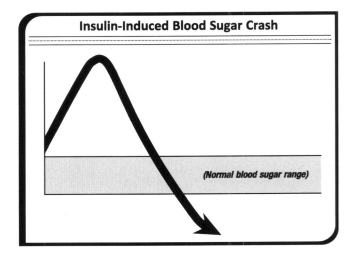

Insulin-Induced Blood Sugar Crash

(Normal blood sugar range)

not buy ten pair? Because you don't need ten pair! Consuming more protein than you need for cellular repair, the immune system, and other bodily functions, will simply lead to fat storage.

Yes, protein can be converted to body fat.

More calories than you can use at a time is too much food regardless of what it is. When carbs are consumed in too large of quantities, the hormone insulin is secreted and drives the storage processes described. Bad news if you're trying to lose body fat. What happens when too much protein is consumed, though? You guessed it; insulin is secreted from the pancreas as well. Granted, we typically won't eat hundreds of grams of protein in one meal—a feat easily performed with carbs—but too much is still too much; it's not free.

It can also be dangerous. I mentioned it already, so I'll let you Google the controversy surrounding high protein intake; I simply suggest getting what you need for good health, easy dieting, lean body mass needs, and high energy levels.

Early low-carb diets suggested you could eat as much fat as you want and life would be grand. If you avoid carbs, nothing else matters, right? Eat a couple pounds of butter a week, as many burgers as you want, but just avoid carbs, and not only would you lose weight, but your cholesterol levels would fall. I don't want to make light of the fact that some people are more carb sensitive and do better by controlling carbs with

> We need to manage carbs to avoid gaining weight. We need to reduce them to lose weight, but carbs are critically important—we can't drop them completely.

a tighter fist. If that's the case, they can eat a little more protein or fat. But, as soon as a meal is sufficient in size, ninety-seven percent of dietary fat is stored as fat.

The first issue of meal dynamics is pure caloric quantity. But, if the thermic potential of protein is up to thirty percent and the thermic potential of carbohydrate is up to thirty percent, why would you consume more dietary fat and risk storing body fat due to a low three-percent thermic potential? Consuming more dietary fat than you can use at a meal results in easy and immediate storage as body fat.

> Consuming more dietary fat than you can use at a meal results in easy and immediate storage as body fat.

Putting it All Together

As a way of organizing this information in your mind, think of two sets of three different energy sources. There are external and internal sources of protein, carbs, and fat. We consume protein, carbs, and fat in the food we eat but we also have stored versions of each. Carbs are stored in our liver and muscle, protein is stored as amino acids in muscle tissue and the liver, and body fat can be stored...everywhere! It isn't a linear process of going from one to the other as a source is used up, but changing percentages of each follow a physiologically predictable pattern. When there is glucose present and entering our blood stream from our diet, we use that first as energy. Carbs in our diet. If we're managing our carbs well, we'll need another source of energy between meals, and true to our body's need for glucose, it will turn to the

> " All three macronutrients have a role, all three are important in the right amounts, and all three can be used in a targeted fashion to maximize their strengths and minimize potential weaknesses.

easiest source possible: liver and muscle glycogen. Stored carbs.

We can only get to body fat once we're managing carbs well and have spent a couple of days working through stockpiled carbs. But, if we're consuming a lot of dietary fat, we'll use that first simply because it's available. That will limit how much body fat we need to use. We have to keep an eye on fat intake—it's not a carb-only issue.

If we have a sufficient amount of dietary protein to provide the amino acids we need—and not too much more—then protein is not a dynamic factor. We're preventing muscle loss and stimulating the metabolism, but it's really the relationship between carbs and fat that helps drive fat loss. All three macronutrients have a role, all three are important in the right amounts, and all three can be used in a targeted fashion to maximize their strengths and minimize potential weaknesses. That is the essence of precise timing and losing body fat as consistently and efficiently as possible.

Back to Metabolic Positioning

I remember a fifty-four-year-old woman who called one day and said, "I've been on diets non-stop for twenty-nine years. I had a total hysterectomy after my last child and could never lose that weight. I know my endocrine system is messed up; I'm afraid I'll never be able to lose this weight. I've never lost more than two pounds on a diet; it's my metabolism—I can't lose anything."

I love a challenge.

I explained metabolic positioning to her during her initial consultation. She lost a couple of pounds her first week. She hit ten pounds. She asked me if it would be possible to lose twenty-five pounds by her fifty-fifth birthday for a vacation she was taking.

Fifteen pounds…

Twenty pounds…

I could barely understand a voicemail from her because she was crying.

Twenty-five pounds.

In six months she had lost forty-five pounds. She reached her pre-pregnancy weight. What was that she said about not being able to lose? The difference was having the right macronutritional profile but also making sure she stayed in the right place metabolically where her body was using body fat as a strong secondary source of energy between meals.

Consistently.

Reducing metabolic science to quick, easy steps isn't always quick or easy. Though our goal is to provide a fast, organized system to get you on your way, take your time and learn how your body works. I guess this paragraph is a subtle apology for dumping so much physiology on you, but it's worth it. Here's one last list to review how you can tap into body fat maximally:

✔ Manage carbs appropriately per meal and per day.

✔ Work through stored carb (glycogen) sources.

✔ Transition to maximal body fat use between meals.

✔ Consume enough protein to maximize the use of amino acids.

✔ Target needs meal by meal to maximize fat loss.

✔ Target needs meal by meal to keep the metabolism blazing.

✔ Be consistent.

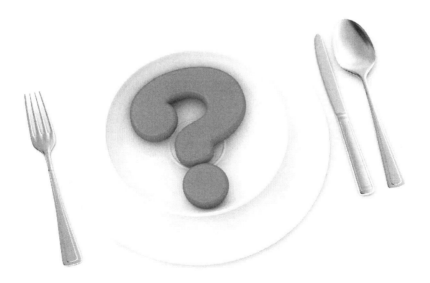

CHAPTER FOUR

Precision Meals

CORE	Protein/Starch
RECOVERY	Protein/Fiber
ANCHOR	Protein/Starch/Fiber
PRE-WORKOUT	Starch-Sugar
POST-WORKOUT	Protein
REPLENISH	Protein/Starch (half serving)

STRUCTURE AND FLEXIBILITY. If weight management is important to you, I would almost advise you to tattoo those words, one on each wrist. You'll be lean and in the cool crowd. Maybe a note on your bathroom mirror will suffice. Most diet plans provide structure—too much structure. It's easy for the designer/author to create a meal plan—a monkey could do it with a couple clicks of the mouse. It's easy for the reader/dieter to utilize a rigid meal plan—they don't have to think. "Just eat this" becomes the game plan and everyone's happy. The problem is that it's a recipe for failure. Most get tripped up right away because life isn't exactly the same every day. Others may end up losing some weight by thoughtlessly eating the same foods—maybe foods they don't even like—but the regain begins as soon as they're bored. Sustainable behavior change comes from new knowledge.

> Sustainable behavior change comes from new knowledge.

Of course, achieving short- or long-term success assumes the structure is even factual and effective. Most plans you'll encounter make it to market not because they're correct, but because they're novel. The sizzle sells the steak and this is a crowded industry—the sizzle keeps growing louder and the claims are becoming more outlandish. Unfortunately, a shiny new marketing spin won't help you. The structure of a diet plan has to be physiologically sound and that means that the interpretation of existing research has to be accurate. One final problem to contend with is that many so-called experts think there is only one such interpretation. There are two levels of flexibility often missed.

Proven metabolic physiology should provide enough structure, but you have to account for genetic body type differences and you have to yield to social flexibility. Every day can pose challenges with eating the same foods or meals. Consider that once you've met your goals, you need to be well-equipped for a life of continued success. That doesn't include feeling forced to eat the same foods every day. You must learn to use flexibility while you're progressing in order to enjoy a lifetime of practical achievement. Permanent means permanent.

Increasing your metabolism to maximal levels requires a macronutrient arrangement and meal format that attains perfection. Almost. Let me define metabolic perfection. The rest of this section will outline specific meals with specific macronutrient combinations at specific times of the day to achieve maximal metabolic stimulation. The good news is that perfection can be achieved with layers of flexibility as long as the options exist.

Now, I promised that we wouldn't put you to sleep. You're about to step into the metabolic transformation arena. Grab some popcorn and get ready for the show!

CORE	Protein/Starch
RECOVERY	Protein/Fiber
ANCHOR	Protein/Starch/Fiber
PRE-WORKOUT	Starch-Sugar
POST-WORKOUT	Protein
REPLENISH	Protein/Starch (half serving)

CHAPTER FIVE

Breakfast

EATING A BIG breakfast has become accepted dogma within most diets. The last food consumed was probably eight to twelve hours earlier and you have a big day ahead. Fuel up! The rationale is logical and still holds water. I just want to make sure you're not eating a couple Belgian waffles with whip cream and washing it down with half a pound of biscuits and gravy. Let's go back to metabolism. By not eating for that long of a stretch, being relatively still, and with your sympathetic nervous system cruising on autopilot, even your body temperature is at least a degree cooler when you wake up. Your metabolism is at a daily low and you don't want to stay there.

Recall thermic potential—consuming food increases metabolism.

You are on a budgeted amount of calories, so breakfast can't be unlimited, but eat something. Too big of a breakfast will still cause a sharp elevation of insulin and possibly create some early lethargy, so this may take a little experimentation. A full serving of carbs will wake up your metabolism and get you moving into your day, but consume too few carbs and you may find that you're behind the hunger curve all day and can't catch up. One challenge can be that typical breakfast foods contain more than a serving. This is one meal where watching labels might be eye opening.

Blood sugar and even liver glycogen might be low from fasting all night, but so are blood nitrogen levels (amino acid content). Reversing this catabolic environment as soon as possible with breakfast is important to retain muscle and spur the metabolism. Studies have shown the importance of protein at breakfast particularly through hunger patterns. Even children who add protein to their breakfast have been noted to eat hundreds of fewer calories per day.

Protein and carbohydrates are recommended at breakfast, but let's talk about a possible deviation. What if you work out in the morning? In that case, I would recommend having your pre- and post-workout meals as specified. Breakfast—being a Core Meal—can then become a mid-morning snack if there is a long gap between your post-workout meal and lunch. The workout will likely create more hunger in the following few hours and it's a good place to support the training. If lunch is only three to four hours away, you might just want to wait and make it a mid-day Anchor Meal.

" Studies have shown the importance of protein at breakfast particularly through hunger patterns.

CORE MEALS
Women

Goal:	Protein 20-25	Carbs 25-30	Fat 5-10	Calories 225-310
OPTION ONE				
½ c. oatmeal (dry measure)	5	27	3	155
¼ oz. chopped nuts	1	1	4	44
3 egg whites	9	0	0	36
¼ c. fat-free cheese	9	1	0	40
Total	**24**	**29**	**7**	**275**
OPTION TWO				
½ whole-grain English muffin	2.5	12	1	67
1 tbsp. peanut butter	4	3	8	100
½ c. fat-free cottage cheese	14	5	0	76
¼ c. blueberries	1	5	0	24
Total	**21.5**	**25**	**9**	**267**
OPTION THREE				
½ c. Greek yogurt (fruit)	12	17	0	116
1 rice cake	1	7	0	32
1 tbsp. almond butter	4	3	8	100
3 hard-boiled egg whites	9	0	0	36
Total	**26**	**27**	**8**	**284**
OPTION FOUR				
1 c. canned pumpkin	2	18	0	80
⅔ scoop vanilla Diet Doc protein	20	3	2	108
¼ oz. candied pecans	0	3	3	39
Total	**22**	**24**	**5**	**227**

OPTION FIVE

½ c. cooked brown rice	2	18	.5	84.5
2 egg whites (boiled or scrambled)	6	0	0	24
1.5 oz. diced chicken breast	11	0	1	53
1 oz. diced tomato or salsa	1	2	0	12
1 oz. avocado	1	3	4.5	56.5
Total	**21**	**23**	**6**	**230**

OPTION SIX

¼ c. black beans	3.5	9	1	59
2 oz. extra-lean ground turkey	12	0	2	66
¼ c. low-fat feta cheese	6	1	4	64
1 low-carb tortilla	5	15	3	107
2 tbsp. salsa	1	2	0	12
Total	**27.5**	**27**	**10**	**308**

OPTION SEVEN

2 slices whole-grain toast	5	30	2	158
3 egg whites	9	0	0	36
2 pieces turkey or veggie bacon	6	0	3	51
1 slice low-fat cheese	5	0	4	60
1 slice tomato	0	1	0	4
Total	**25**	**31**	**9**	**262**

OPTION EIGHT

½ c. high-fiber cereal	6	22	.5	116.5
½ c. skim milk	4	5.5	0	38
½ oz. slivered almonds	3	3	6	78
4 egg whites	12	0	0	48
Totals	**25**	**30.5**	**6.5**	**280.5**

OPTION NINE

¾ c. fat-free cottage cheese	21	7.5	0	114
1 oz. low-fat granola	3	15	7.5	139.5
Totals	**24**	**22.5**	**7.5**	**253.5**

	Protein	Carbs	Fat	Calories
1 small protein bar	13	23	7	207
½ c. plain Greek yogurt	12	5	0	68
Total	**25**	**28**	**7**	**275**

CORE MEALS

Men

Goal:	Protein 30-35	Carbs 30-35	Fat 10-15	Calories 330-415
OPTION ONE				
½ c. oatmeal (dry measure)	5	27	3	155
½ oz. walnuts	3	3	10	114
1 oz. blueberries	0	4	0	16
5 egg whites	15	0	0	60
¼ c. fat-free cheese	9	1	0	40
Total	**32**	**35**	**13**	**385**
OPTION TWO				
1 whole-grain English muffin	6	22	1	121
1 tbsp. peanut butter	4	3	8	100
⅔ c. fat-free cottage cheese	18.5	6	0	98
1 oz. diced tomatoes	0	1	0	4
1 oz. avocado	1	3	4.5	56.5
Total	**29.5**	**35**	**13.5**	**379.5**
OPTION THREE				
½ c. Greek yogurt (fruit)	12	17	0	116
¼ c. oatmeal (dry measure)	2.5	13	1.5	75.5
1 tsp. flax seed oil	0	0	5	45
¾ scoop vanilla Diet Doc protein	21	3	2	116
Total	**36.5**	**33**	**8.5**	**352.5**

OPTION FOUR

1 c. canned pumpkin	2	18	0	80
¾ scoop vanilla Diet Doc protein	21	3	2	116
½ oz. candied pecans	.5	6	5.5	75.5
¼ c. fat-free cottage cheese	7	2.5	0	38
Total	**30.5**	**29.5**	**7.5**	**309.5**

OPTION FIVE

½ c. cooked brown rice	2	18	.5	84.5
½ c. skim milk	4	5.5	0	38
¾ scoop vanilla Diet Doc protein	21	3	2	116
⅓ oz. pistachios	2	3	5	65
Cinnamon	0	0	0	0
Total	**29**	**29.5**	**7.5**	**303.5**

OPTION SIX

¼ c. black beans	3.5	9	1	59
¼ c. low-fat cheddar cheese	6	1	4	64
1 low-carb tortilla	5	15	3	107
2 tbsp. salsa	1	2	0	12
2 egg whites	6	0	0	24
1 oz. diced chicken	7	0	1	37
1 oz. avocado	1	3	4.5	56.5
1 tbsp. fat-free sour cream	1	2	0	12
Total	**30.5**	**32**	**13.5**	**371.5**

Scramble egg whites and mix in beans and chicken to warm. Spoon into a crisped tortilla and sprinkle with cheese. Top with salsa, avocado, and sour cream.

OPTION SEVEN

2 slices whole-grain toast	5	30	2	158
4 egg whites	12	0	0	48
1 piece turkey or veggie bacon	4	0	5	61
2 slices fat-free pepper jack cheese	10	2	0	48
½ oz. almonds	3	3	7	87
Total	**21**	**28**	**8**	**402**

OPTION EIGHT

5 oz. sweet potato	3	29	1	137
¾ scoop vanilla Diet Doc protein	21	3	2	116
1 tsp. flax seed oil	0	0	5	45
3 egg whites	9	0	0	36
Totals	**33**	**32**	**8**	**334**

Mix protein & flax seed oil with warm, mashed sweet potato; cook egg whites to have on the side, or scramble and fold into sweet potato mixture.

OPTION NINE

1 tortilla wrap	5	20	4	136
3 oz. lean turkey or beef	18	0	3	99
½ oz. low-fat cheese	5	0	4	56
¼ c. mushrooms	2	2	0	16
¼ c. diced tomatoes	1	4	0	20
1 c. broccoli	1	4	0	20
Totals	**30**	**30**	**11**	**339**

Cook egg whites omelet style with mushrooms and broccoli. Fold into tortilla with cheese. Top with diced tomatoes and avocado.

OPTION TEN

¼ c. high-fiber cereal	3	11	0	56
½ c. blueberries	2	5.5	0	36
1 c. low-fat cottage cheese	28	8	2.5	166.5
1 tbsp. peanut butter	4	3	8	100
Total	**35**	**31**	**10.5**	**378.5**

CORE	Protein/Starch
RECOVERY	Protein/Fiber
ANCHOR	Protein/Starch/Fiber
PRE-WORKOUT	Starch-Sugar
POST-WORKOUT	Protein
REPLENISH	Protein/Starch (half serving)

CHAPTER SIX

Lunch

I HAVEN'T BEEN too subtle explaining that low-carb diets are a titanic failure for long-term weight management. Nothing will suppress your metabolism faster, cause lean body mass loss, and set you up for rapid fat regain like dropping carbs too low. Due to body type differences, though, some people do have to consume lower amounts of carbs than others—it's a point of management, not extremism. When trying to lose body fat, it can be a good idea through the course of a day to have spans where carbs are low, as long as too much time doesn't pass. It's a delicate dance between doing what's right to keep your metabolism high yet tapping into body fat reserves to keep losing.

> There is a dynamic tension between needing to reduce carbs to lose, and having enough carbs to keep metabolic processes stimulated.

Carbs have to be low enough to progressively work through stored glycogen levels in your body to ultimately use higher percentages of body fat for energy. There is a dynamic tension between reducing carbs to lose, and having enough carbs to keep metabolic processes stimulated. It can be a hard concept to understand, but it's a central metabolic truth. Timing is everything. There are times it is safe, proper, and necessary to reduce carbs through the day, but there are times you need a surge of energy provided by carbohydrate. Those surges not only provide needed energy, but also sharp metabolic boosts and protection against muscle loss.

One of the two typically larger meals of the day—lunch and dinner—should be a place where starchy carbs are sacrificed to use at more important times. Since meals will be eaten often enough to reduce hunger, and targeted carb intake is the name of the game, a couple meals consumed with lower starch content will enhance fat loss considerably. Between meals—once digestion and assimilation is complete—an incremental increase in stored fat usage will occur. When a meal doesn't contain a lot of carbohydrate, the return to body fat as an energy source can happen more quickly.

We leave it as a personal choice whether dinner or lunch is selected to be an Anchor Meal with protein, a starchy carbohydrate (or half a serving), and a fibrous carbohydrate. It doesn't even have to remain a constant through the diet—it can change day to day as schedules shift. Most may find that the evening meal works better as a larger, more complete meal so the night hours are set up for less hunger. During the day, most are busy with work and it can be easier to make lunch a lighter meal. Consider the circumstance described in the last chapter where a morning workout may provide enough food in the pre- and post-workout meals to make it to lunch without eating again. By lunch you may be hungry enough to make it your Anchor Meal with a starchy carb source. Changing circumstances can alter which decision is best. The choice is yours—it's another key example of how flexibility can make or break a sustainable diet plan.

RECOVERY MEALS
Women

Goal:	Protein 20-25	Carbs 10-15	Fat 5-10	Calories 165-250
OPTION ONE				
2.5 oz. chicken breast	17.5	0	2.5	94.5
2 c. of green beans	2	10	0	48
½ oz. low-fat feta cheese	2	1	3	39
Small salad, 1 tbsp. balsamic	1.5	3.5	3.5	51.5
(1 c. spinach, 1 oz. tomato, 1 oz. cucumber)				
Total	**22.5**	**14.5**	**9**	**233**
OPTION TWO				
½ whole-grain English muffin	2.5	12	1	67
1 can of tuna in water	22	0	1	97
1 oz. avocado	1	3	4.5	56.5
Total	**25.5**	**15**	**6.5**	**220.5**
OPTION THREE				
2 oz. lean ground turkey	14	0	3	83
¼ c. black beans	3.5	9	0	50
⅓ oz. fat-free mozzarella	3	0	0	12
1 tbsp. light sour cream	2	1	2	56.5
1 tbsp. salsa, ¼ c shredded lettuce	0	3	0	12
Total	**22.5**	**13**	**5**	**207**

OPTION FOUR

3 oz. salmon	21	0	6	138
1 c. asparagus	2	4	0	24
¼ c. cooked brown rice	1	9	.5	44.5
Total	**25**	**13**	**6.5**	**206.5**

OPTION FIVE

Low-carb pita	7	10	1.5	81.5
2 oz. chicken breast	14	0	2	74
1 tbsp. hummus	2	2	2.5	38.5
Lettuce leaf and tomato slice	1	2	0	12
Total	**24**	**14**	**6**	**206**

OPTION SIX

½ c. fat-free cottage cheese	13	5	0	72
½ c. blueberries	0	6	0	24
⅓ oz. walnuts	1	1.5	6	64
1.5 oz. chicken breast	10	0	1.5	53.5
Lettuce leaf and tomato slice	1	2	0	12
Total	**27.5**	**27**	**8**	**225.5**

OPTION SEVEN

1 vegetarian burger patty	18	8	1	113
1 tbsp. hummus	1.5	2	3.5	45.5
1 c. steamed broccoli	1	4	0	20
1 tsp. flax oil	0	0	5	45
Total	**20.5**	**14**	**9.5**	**223.5**

OPTION EIGHT

1 corn tostada shell	2	8	.5	44.5
2 oz. white fish or shrimp	14	0	2	74
½ oz. low-fat cheese	5	0	2.5	42.5
2 tbsp. salsa	0	4	0	16
1 tbsp. light sour cream	2	1	2	30
Totals	**23**	**13**	**7**	**207**

OPTION NINE

	Protein	Carbs	Fat	Calories
½ c. butternut squash (3 ½ oz.)	1	10.5	0	46
½ oz. low-fat cheese	5	0	2.5	42.5
3 oz. sirloin	18	0	6	126
Totals	**24**	**10.5**	**8.5**	**214**

OPTION TEN

	Protein	Carbs	Fat	Calories
1 slice whole-wheat toast	2	15	1	77
½ can tuna in water	11	0	1	53
1 oz. cheese	10	0	6	94
1 tbsp. fat-free mayo	0	2	0	8
Total	**23**	**17**	**8**	**232**

Add spices to taste.

RECOVERY MEALS

Men

	Protein	Carbs	Fat	Calories
Goal:	**35-40**	**15-20**	**10-15**	**290-375**

OPTION ONE

	Protein	Carbs	Fat	Calories
3 oz. chicken breast	21	0	3	90
1 oz. fat-free cheese	9	2	0	44
1 c. fresh spinach	2	3	0	20
½ oz. walnuts	3	3	10	114
1 c. strawberries	0	11	0	44
1 tbsp. low-fat dressing	0	1	1	13
Total	**35**	**20**	**14**	**325**

OPTION TWO

	Protein	Carbs	Fat	Calories
1 whole-grain English muffin	5	24	2	134
1 can of tuna in water	22	0	1	97
1 oz. avocado	1	3	4.5	56.5
1 c. lettuce	0	2	0	4
1 oz. diced tomato	0	.5	0	2
2 boiled egg whites	6	0	0	24
Total	**34**	**29.5**	**7.5**	**317.5**

OPTION THREE

½ c. plain Greek yogurt	12	5	0	68
¼ c. high-fiber cereal	3	11	1	65
½ tsp. flax seed oil	0	0	5	54
¾ scoop vanilla Diet Doc protein	21	3	2	116
Total	**36**	**19**	**8**	**303**

OPTION FOUR

3 oz. extra-lean ground beef	21	0	3	90
¼ c. black beans	3.5	9	0	50
1 tbsp. salsa	1	2	0	12
¼ c. plain Greek yogurt	6	3	0	36
3 oz. lettuce	1	3	0	16
1 oz. cheese	7	2	6	90
Total	**39.5**	**19**	**9**	**294**

OPTION FIVE

Low-carb pita	7	10	1.5	81.5
2 oz. chicken breast	14	0	2	74
1 serving turkey pepperoni	9	0	4.5	76.5
¼ c. mozzarella cheese	10	2	5	93
1 oz. mushroom	1	1	0	8
Total	**41**	**13**	**13**	**333**

Pita Pizza: Top pita with sauce, cheese, and meat. Bake on rack to desired crispness.

OPTION SIX

½ scoop Diet Doc Protein	10.5	3	2	72
¾ c. plain Greek yogurt	17.5	7	0	98
¼ c. blueberries	1	4	0	20
1 oz. almonds	6	6	14	174
Total	**35**	**20**	**16**	**364**

OPTION SEVEN

2 vegetarian burger patties	36	16	2	226
2 tbsp. hummus	3	4	7	91
Total	**39**	**20**	**9**	**317**

OPTION EIGHT

2 hard corn tortilla shells	3	16	6	130
4 oz. tilapia	28	0	2	130
¼ c. shredded cabbage	0	1	0	4
1 oz. low-fat shredded cheddar	9	0	5	81
Totals	**40**	**17**	**13**	**342**

OPTION NINE

1 tortilla wrap	9	17	2.5	126.5
3.5 oz. turkey	24	0	3	123
1 oz. cheese	5	0	9	101
1 leaf lettuce	0	1	0	4
1 dill pickle	0	2	0	8
1 tbsp. mustard	0	0	0	0
Totals	**38**	**20**	**14.5**	**362.5**

OPTION TEN

½ English muffin	2.5	13	.5	66.5
1 tbsp. peanut butter	4	3	8	100
¼ c. sliced apples (1 oz.)	2	4	0	24
4 oz. chicken breast	28	0	4	148
Total	**36.5**	**20**	**12.5**	**338.5**

CHAPTER SEVEN

Dinner

CORE	Protein/Starch
RECOVERY	Protein/Fiber
ANCHOR	Protein/Starch/Fiber
PRE-WORKOUT	Starch-Sugar
POST-WORKOUT	Protein
REPLENISH	Protein/Starch (half serving)

I MENTIONED THIS in the previous chapter, but let me reiterate that dinner is a pivotal point in the day. Many of us feel a profound shift when the work day is complete and we're transitioning to home life. A sense of relief and a let down from a fast pace and stress can often marry food to an expectation—even subconsciously—of a relaxing evening. Some European countries still practice the art of long family dinners for that very reason. That's why we consider this a good place for your Anchor Meal; we understand that this meal can be a set-up for a successful evening. If too little is eaten, it may trigger uncontrolled snacking at night—a common breakdown of weight-loss progress.

Whether you choose to have a complete serving of starchy carbohydrates, or half (per the choice to flip lunch and dinner guidelines), there will still be a fibrous carb source added to protein to make it a complete meal. This can ensure stability for the rest of the evening. Those who stay up late may need to take advantage of the Replenish Meal to make it to bedtime without a lot of hunger.

I'm willing to guess that evenings don't look the same for everyone. If your family dinner scene doesn't include mom with an apron shuttling a five-course meal to the table, dad at the head of the table in a suit, and the children sitting quietly with cloth napkins folded in their laps, welcome to the club. A typical night for me involves sprinting out of the office to a ball field or school event, either grabbing something on the way, my wife meeting me there with my dinner, or just waiting until I eventually get home. These are scenarios we all have to think through and plan for if we're going to be successful in losing weight and maintaining good health. This is real life.

I wrote this chapter in a hotel lobby. My son and I were at a travel-team baseball tournament and a couple meals had to be eaten in restaurants. As a bit of a rule, I try to eat just one meal out per day and pack the rest of my food when traveling. Dried fruit, protein powder, almonds, protein bars, and other easy-to-carry foods make it possible. My eight-year-old daughter helped me pack it; she manned the digital scale to make sure the snacks were the appropriate serving size. Not a bad bit of parental modeling, eh?

We ate an early dinner in a buffet-style restaurant—the scourge of the Midwest—and I observed something I think you can relate to. Most of the adults started out with a salad, and most of the salads have a high volume of ingredients that disqualify them as diet friendly. Still, the parents felt that they're eating healthy. The entrée trip was next and two-to-three times a normal protein intake was brought back from the kill. At home, would you eat three different types of meat? Same story with starchy carbs: because the array of choices was vast, plates were piled high. The rationalization started. "I probably shouldn't have any dessert, but…"

That, dear reader, is the primary reason that a third of adults are obese. It may not be a buffet every day, but that same decision-making process is made over and over and over. At a drive-through, do you need two or three pieces of cheese on a half-pound burger with a quarter-cup of mayo? How many grams of fat are in those fries? At a friend's house, do you need a serving of everything; will they really be offended if you don't? When a coworker brings doughnuts to work, is it an automatic grab? I call this opportunity-based failure because every time our normal schedule is interrupted with an opportunity to "cheat," how often do we take it? It has to become our new norm to stop, think, and then decide. Maybe you can enjoy something a little off plan by just adjusting other meals in your day, or maybe this particular meal or snack is one that just isn't worth the disruption. It's your choice.

I have learned in virtually every situation to make that choice. *Will I eat healthy or is this meal worth the added body fat I know it will cause?* When I stop at a drive-through for lunch or dinner, all of the fast-food places around my office know it's me when they hear, "I'll have a number thirteen, sandwich only, no cheese, no mayo." Once you start making decisions based on your goals, you'll see that it's a powerful victory regarding control. Stop and think.

> It has to become our new norm to stop, think, and then decide.

ANCHOR MEALS

Women

Goal:	Protein 15-20	Carbs 30-35	Fat 0-5	Calories 180-265
OPTION ONE				
8 slices turkey pepperoni	4	0	3	43
1 English muffin	5	24	1	125
¼ c. marinara	1	4	1	29
¼ c. fat-free mozzarella cheese	9	2	0	44
3 oz. salad with fat-free dressing	1	5	0	24
Total	**20**	**35**	**5**	**265**

English muffin pizzas: split muffin and top with marinara, cheese, and pepperoni. Broil until cheese has browned. Serve with a side salad.

OPTION TWO

2 oz. lean beef	12	0	4	84
1 slice fat-free cheese	4	3	0	28
1 slice whole-grain toast	2	15	.5	72.5
2 oz. sweet potato	1	13	0	56
Total	19	31	4.5	240.5

OPTION THREE

2 oz. sirloin	16	0	4	90
2 c. broccoli	2	8	0	40
3 oz. potato	1.5	20	0	86
Total	19.5	28	4	216

OPTION FOUR

½ c. oatmeal (dry measure)	5	27	3	155
¼ c. pumpkin	1	4.5	0	22
½ scoop vanilla Diet Doc protein	14	2	1.5	77.5
Total	20	33.5	4.5	254.5

OPTION FIVE

1.5 oz. chicken breast	10	0	1.5	53.5
½ oz. shredded fat-free cheddar	4.5	1	0	22
2 tbsp. salsa	0	2	0	8
¼ c. black beans	3.5	9	0	50
1 serving baked tortilla chips	3	22	2	118
Total	21	34	3.5	251.5

OPTION SIX

2 oz. shrimp	12	0	1	57
½ c. rice	2	22	1	105
½ oz. fat-free cheese	4.5	1	0	22
1 oz. spinach & 1 oz. tomato	2	4	0	24
2 oz. strawberries	0	4	0	14
1 tbsp. fat-free balsamic	0	1	2	22
Total	20.5	32	4	244

OPTION SEVEN

½ c. fat-free cottage cheese	14	5	0	76
¼ c. diced tomato	1	2	0	12
1 oz. cucumber	0	1	0	4
½ oz. pinto beans	1.5	3.5	0	20
1 serving pita chips	3	19	5	133
Total	**19.5**	**30.5**	**5**	**245**

OPTION EIGHT

1 small baked potato (5 oz.)	3	27	.5	124.5
½ c. low-fat cottage cheese	14	5	2.5	98.5
¼ c. pizza sauce	1	2	.5	16.5
Totals	**18**	**34**	**3.5**	**239.5**

Melt cottage cheese on a warm potato and top with pizza or marinara sauce.

OPTION NINE

1 whole-grain wrap	9	17	2.5	126.5
Lettuce leaf	0	2	0	8
¼ c. cooked white rice	1	11	0	48
1 oz. chicken breast	7	0	1	37
Totals	**17**	**30**	**3.5**	**219.5**

OPTION TEN

1 serving pretzels	3	21	0	96
2 oz. deli turkey	12	0	2	66
1 sliced small apple (3.5 oz.)	.5	14	0	58
Total	**15.5**	**35**	**2**	**220**

ANCHOR MEALS

Men

	Protein	Carbs	Fat	Calories
Goal:	30-35	45-50	5-10	345-430
OPTION ONE				
3 oz. sirloin strips	24	0	6	150
¾ c. rice	3	33	1	153
1 c. broccoli	1	4	0	20
2 oz. mushroom	1	2	0	12
3 oz. sliced red pepper	1	7	0	32
1 tbsp. soy sauce	0	0	0	0
Total	**30**	**46**	**7**	**367**
OPTION TWO				
1.5 oz. chicken	10	0	1.5	53.5
½ c. fat-free refried beans	8	19	0	108
1 whole-grain tortilla	6	24	3	147
1 oz. fat-free shredded cheddar	9	2	0	44
1 c. shredded lettuce	0	2	0	8
2 tbsp. salsa	0	2	0	8
Total	**35**	**49**	**4.5**	**368.5**
OPTION THREE				
1 c. skim milk	8	11	0	76
1 c. cereal	2	23	0	100
¼ c. blueberries	0	4	0	16
¾ scoop vanilla Diet Doc protein	21	3	2	116
1 tbsp. flax seeds	2	1	4	48
Total	**33**	**43**	**6**	**356**

OPTION FOUR

½ c. oatmeal (dry measure)	5	27	3	155
½ c. fat-free cottage cheese	14	5	0	76
½ scoop vanilla Diet Doc protein	14	2	1.5	77.5
½ c. peaches	1	8	.5	40.5
Total	**34**	**42**	**5**	**349**

Cook oats; add other ingredients (or use raw oats like granola).

OPTION FIVE

4 oz. shrimp	28	0	3	139
1 tostada shell	1	7	2	50
1 oz. fat-free feta cheese	7	0	0	28
1 c. shredded lettuce	0	2	0	8
¾ c. Spanish rice	3	35	5	197
Total	**39**	**44**	**10**	**422**

OPTION SIX

4 oz. chicken breast	28	0	4	148
½ c. chunky marinara	3	13	3	91
1 c. butternut squash	2	20	0	88
3 oz. sautéed onions/zucchini	2	10	2	66
Total	**35**	**43**	**9**	**393**

OPTION SEVEN

4 oz. salmon	24	0	8	168
1 c. cooked rice noodles	2	44	.5	188.5
1 c. broccoli	1	4	0	20
1 tbsp. parmesan cheese	2	0	1.5	21.5
Total	**29**	**48**	**10**	**398**

OPTION EIGHT

1 medium potato (6 oz.)	4	34	0	152
3.5 oz. sirloin	30	0	6.5	178.5
1 c. broccoli	1	4	0	20
⅓ c. unsweetened applesauce	0	9	0	36
Totals	**35**	**47**	**6.5**	**386.5**

OPTION NINE

2 oz. pasta (uncooked weight)	7	41	1	201
1 can tuna in water	22	0	2	106
3 oz. raw spinach	3	2	0	20
½ oz. low-fat cheese	2	2	1.5	29.5
Totals	**34**	**45**	**4.5**	**356.5**

OPTION TEN

1 flour tortilla	5	35	2	178
¼ c. kernel corn	1.5	9	0	42
1 oz. low-fat shredded cheddar	9	0	5	81
2.5 oz. extra-lean ground turkey	17	0	2.5	90.5
Total	**32.5**	**44**	**9.5**	**391.5**

CORE	Protein/Starch
RECOVERY	Protein/Fiber
ANCHOR	Protein/Starch/Fiber
PRE-WORKOUT	Starch-Sugar
POST-WORKOUT	Protein
REPLENISH	Protein/Starch (half serving)

CHAPTER EIGHT

Pre-Workout & Post-Workout Snacks

SOME FITNESS MAGAZINES are starting to report actual studies on pre- and post-training nutrition needs, but we're facing over fifty years of opinion and myth. You might still subscribe to the must-exercise-in-the-morning-on-an-empty-stomach rule, but it's time to let it go. The thought process is that when blood sugar and liver glycogen levels are low—no food while sleeping—the body will immediately use body fat as a greater part of energy use. That is actually true, but you also risk using more amino acids from muscle (muscle loss), and that's not the entire metabolic story.

If you consume a small amount of carbs first, you'll have a much stronger, more effective cardio session. More calories are likely to be burned, more calories will be used during the subsequent couple of hours (even at rest), risk of lean body mass loss is reduced, and studies show collectively that more body fat loss occurs compared to fasted cardio. Be careful to use a small amount of carbs—just enough to prime the pump.

Carbs before cardio or training are important whether it's first thing in the morning or mid-afternoon. Time the pre-workout snack fifteen- to sixty-minutes prior to training. In terms of weight

training or functional training, you'll be glad you have that fuel for energy so that the workout is productive enough to push forward with progress.

One of the biggest post-workout concerns is hormonal in nature. Cortisol levels will be high, and without the proper nutritional support, the threat of losing muscle and driving the body into a state of adrenal fatigue is greater. Studies show that consuming protein immediately after training will arrest this process. If carbs are added to this meal, staving off catabolism isn't the only benefit; recovery, strength gains, and muscle growth can occur at higher rates. Don't let that convince you that carbs have to be consumed post-workout, though. Protein is necessary—carbs are a luxury. The next meal or two will be your back up for carbs. If burning body fat is your primary goal, stick with protein alone.

Because you have the choice of when you'll work out, you should be concerned how the pre- and post-training snacks affect the other meals. As I mentioned previously, if you train in the morning, the pre- and post-workout meals may be all you need until lunch if there isn't a long span of time between the post-workout meal and lunch. If there is too much time, you can simply have a Core Meal later in the morning as a snack. Be logical with timing, but also pay attention to hunger levels.

If you train after work, you may have the pre- and post-workout meals plus dinner a little later, eliminating the need for the Replenish Snack. That snack could be used as a morning snack if needed.

Flexibility. I told you it's a big deal.

PRE-WORKOUT MEALS
Women

Goal:	Protein 0-5	Carbs 15-20	Fat 0-5	Calories 60-145
OPTION ONE				
1 rice cake	1	7	0	32
1 tbsp. jam	0	7	0	28
1 tsp. peanut butter	1	1	3	35
Total	**2**	**15**	**3**	**95**
OPTION TWO				
5 low-fat crackers	1	15	1.5	77.5
Total	**1**	**15**	**1.5**	**77.5**
OPTION THREE				
½ small protein bar	4.5	13	3	97
Total	**4.5**	**13**	**3**	**97**
OPTION FOUR				
½ banana	1	15	0	64
1 tsp. peanut butter	1	1	3	35
Total	**2**	**16**	**3**	**99**
OPTION FIVE				
¼ c. oats	2.5	13	1.5	75.5
2 oz. blueberries	0	7	0	28
Total	**2.5**	**20**	**1.5**	**104**

OPTION SIX

6 pita chips	2	12	3	83
Total	**2**	**12**	**3**	**83**

OPTION SEVEN

¼ c. oats	2.5	13	1.5	75.5
1 tsp. almond butter	1	1	3	35
½ oz. canned pumpkin	0	4	0	16
Totals	**3.5**	**18**	**4.5**	**126.5**

Add vanilla extract, cinnamon, stevia, and/or pumpkin pie spice to taste.

OPTION EIGHT

2 chocolate kisses	1	6	3	55
1 flavored rice cake	1	12	0	52
Totals	**2**	**18**	**3**	**107**

OPTION NINE

1 light fat-free yogurt	5	21	0	104
½ tsp. flax seed oil	0	0	3	27
Totals	**5**	**21**	**3**	**131**

OPTION TEN

¾ c. mixed fruit (5 ounces)	1	16	0	68
2 tbsp. Greek yogurt	3	2	0	20
¼ oz. chopped nuts	1	1	4	53
Total	**5**	**19**	**4**	**141**

POST-WORKOUT MEALS
Women

Goal:	Protein 15-20	Carbs 5-10	Fat 0-5	Calories 80-165

OPTION ONE

½ scoop Diet Doc protein	14	2	1.5	77.5
1/8 serving high-fiber cereal	1.5	5.5	.5	32.5
Total	**15.5**	**7.5**	**2.5**	**110**

OPTION TWO

½ cup fat-free cottage cheese	14	5	0	76
2 oz. strawberries	1	4.5	0	22
1 tsp. flax seed oil	0	0	5	45
Total	**15**	**9.5**	**5**	**143**

OPTION THREE

½ scoop Diet Doc protein	14	2	1.5	77.5
1 rice cake	1	7	0	32
Total	**15**	**9**	**1.5**	**109.5**

OPTION FOUR

4 egg whites	12	0	0	48
1 low-carb tortilla	5	10	3	87
Total	**17**	**10**	**3**	**135**

OPTION FIVE

½ c. plain Greek yogurt	12.5	4.5	0	68
1 oz. blueberries	0	3.5	0	14
¼ oz. chopped nuts	1	1	4	44
Total	**13.5**	**9**	**4**	**126**

OPTION SIX

½ c. skim milk	4	5.5	0	38
⅓ scoop Diet Doc protein	9	1	1	49
Total	**13**	**6.5**	**1**	**87**

OPTION SEVEN

5 egg whites	15	0	0	60
1 tbsp. pumpkin	0	1.5	0	6
1/8 c. oatmeal (dry measure)	1	6.5	1	40
1 tsp. almond butter	1	1	3	35
Total	**17**	**9**	**4**	**141**

Mix first 3 ingredients and cook like a pancake. Spread with almond butter.

OPTION EIGHT

	Protein	Carbs	Fat	Calories
2.5 oz. lean ground turkey	17	0	2.5	90.5
1 small corn tortilla	2.5	8	2	60
Totals	**19.5**	**8**	**4.5**	**150.5**

OPTION NINE

	Protein	Carbs	Fat	Calories
2 oz. extra-lean ground beef	12	0	2	66
½ oz. low-fat cheese	2	2	1.5	29.5
2 oz. mushrooms	2	2	0	16
3 oz. broccoli	1	4	0	20
Totals	**17**	**8**	**3.5**	**131.5**

OPTION TEN

	Protein	Carbs	Fat	Calories
¼ banana	0	7	0	28
½ scoop Diet Doc protein	14	2	1.5	77.5
Total	**14**	**9**	**1.5**	**105.5**

PRE-WORKOUT MEALS

Men

Goal:	Protein 0-5	Carbs 25-30	Fat 0-5	Calories 100-185

OPTION ONE

	Protein	Carbs	Fat	Calories
2 rice cakes	2	14	0	64
2 tbsp. jam	0	14	0	56
½ tbsp. peanut butter	2	3	4	56
Total	**4**	**31**	**4**	**176**

OPTION TWO

	Protein	Carbs	Fat	Calories
½ c. oatmeal (dry measure)	5	27	3	155
Total	**5**	**27**	**3**	**155**

OPTION THREE

	Protein	Carbs	Fat	Calories
1 snack-size peanut butter cup	2	10	5	33
1 rice cake	1	7	0	32
½ banana	0	15	0	60
Total	**3**	**32**	**5**	**125**

OPTION FOUR

1 c. diced melon	1	12	0	52
2 oz. low-fat yogurt	2	11	1	61
½ oz. granola	2	7	3	63
Total	**5**	**30**	**4**	**176**

OPTION FIVE

¼ c. oats (dry measure)	2.5	13	1.5	75.5
2 oz. blueberries	0	7	0	28
Total	**2.5**	**20**	**1.5**	**104**

OPTION SIX

12 pita chips	4	24	6	166
Total	**4**	**24**	**6**	**166**

OPTION SEVEN

⅓ c. oats (dry measure)	3	18	2	102
1 tsp. flax oil	0	0	3	27
1 oz. canned pumpkin	0	7.5	0	30
Totals	**3**	**25.5**	**5**	**159**

Add vanilla extract, cinnamon, stevia, and/or pumpkin pie spice to taste.

OPTION EIGHT

1 medium banana (4 oz.)	1	27	.5	116.5
½ tbsp. peanut butter	2	1.5	4	50
Totals	**3**	**28.5**	**4.5**	**166.5**

OPTION NINE

Granola bar	5	24	2	134
Total	**5**	**24**	**2**	**134**

OPTION TEN

1 c. mixed fruit (7 oz.)	1	21	0	88
2 tbsp. Greek yogurt	3	2	0	20
1 tsp. peanut butter	1	1	3	35
Total	**5**	**24**	**3**	**143**

POST-WORKOUT MEALS

Men

Goal:	Protein 20-25	Carbs 10-15	Fat 0-5	Calories 120-205
OPTION ONE				
¾ scoop Diet Doc protein	21	3	2	116
1 rice cake	1	7	0	32
Total	**22**	**10**	**2**	**148**
OPTION TWO				
½ c. fat-free cottage cheese	14	5	0	76
2 oz. strawberries	1	4.5	0	22
1 tsp. flax seed oil	0	0	5	54
Total	**15**	**9.5**	**6**	**143**
OPTION THREE				
3 oz. chicken breast	21	0	3	111
½ mini bagel	2.5	11	1	63
Total	**23.5**	**11**	**4**	**174**
OPTION FOUR				
4 egg whites	12	0	0	48
1 slice fat-free cheese	6	2	0	32
1 low-carb tortilla	5	10	3	87
Total	**23**	**12**	**3**	**167**
OPTION FIVE				
½ c. plain Greek yogurt	12.5	4.5	0	68
1 oz. blueberries	0	3.5	0	14
1 tsp. flax seed oil	0	0	5	45
⅓ scoop Diet Doc protein	9	1	1	49
Total	**21.5**	**9**	**6**	**176**

OPTION SIX

½ c. skim milk	4	5.5	0	38
¾ scoop Diet Doc protein	21	3	2	114
Total	**25**	**8.5**	**2**	**152**

OPTION SEVEN

6 egg whites	18	0	0	72
1 tbsp. pumpkin	0	1.5	0	6
¼ c. oatmeal (dry measure)	2.5	13	1.5	75.5
1 tsp. almond butter	1	1	3	28
Totals	**21.5**	**15.5**	**4.5**	**179.5**

Add vanilla extract, cinnamon, and/or pumpkin pie spice to taste. Mix first 3 ingredients and cook like a pancake. Spread with almond butter.

OPTION EIGHT

½ sandwich thin	2.5	12	1	67
2.5 lean deli meat	17	0	2.5	90.5
Totals	**19.5**	**12**	**3.5**	**157.5**

OPTION NINE

½ serving pita chips	1.5	9	2.5	64.5
7 boiled/chopped egg whites	21	0	0	84
Total	**22.5**	**9**	**2.5**	**148.5**

Add mustard to taste—egg salad.

OPTION TEN

4 oz. extra-lean ground beef	24	0	4	132
¼ c. cooked white rice	1	11	0	48
Total	**25**	**11**	**4**	**180**

CHAPTER NINE

Replenish Snack

CORE	Protein/Starch
RECOVERY	Protein/Fiber
ANCHOR	Protein/Starch/Fiber
PRE-WORKOUT	Starch-Sugar
POST-WORKOUT	Protein
REPLENISH	Protein/Starch (half serving)

THIS SNACK APPEARS at the end of the day on the suggested schedule for those who eat an early dinner and may need a little boost in the late evening. You can think of this as a roving rescue—or emergency—snack. If you don't need it during the evening, use it anywhere in the day you need the energy or hunger relief. Four meals/snacks already include protein; this would make the fifth. The extra protein will enhance recovery from training and can assist with blood sugar stabilization and hunger control any time of the day that you consume it.

A quick, easy replenish snack can also be a protein shake during the day. If you want something more substantial as an evening snack, you might consider an egg white omelet or a chicken breast with a condiment like salsa. A moderate serving of protein, with a small amount of carbohydrate, is the premise of the Replenish Snack.

REPLENISH MEALS

Women

Goal:	Protein 0-5	Carbs 10-15	Fat 0-5	Calories 40-125
OPTION ONE				
1 slice light bread	2	10	1	57
½ tbsp. peanut butter	2	1.5	4	50
Total	**4**	**11.5**	**5**	**107**
OPTION TWO				
½ banana	0	14.5	0	58
½ tbsp. peanut butter	2	1.5	4	50
Total	**2**	**16**	**4**	**108**

OPTION THREE

2 oz. grapes	.5	10	0	42
8 almonds	2	2	5	61
Total	**2.5**	**12**	**5**	**103**

OPTION FOUR

Granola bar	2	15	3	95
Total	**2**	**15**	**3**	**95**

OPTION FIVE

½ light English muffin	2.5	12	.5	62.5
1 tbsp. low-fat cream cheese	2	1	3	39
Slice tomato	1	1	0	8
Total	**5.5**	**14**	**3.5**	**109.5**

OPTION SIX

5 pita chips	1	10	2.5	66.5
½ oz. low-fat cheese	2	1	1.5	25.5
Total	**3**	**11**	**4**	**92**

OPTION SEVEN

½ apple	0	11	0	44
1 piece string cheese	5	0	2	38
Total	**5**	**11**	**2**	**82**

OPTION EIGHT

5 low fat crackers	1.5	10	2.5	68.5
1 tbsp. hummus	2	2.5	2	36
Totals	**3.5**	**12.5**	**4.5**	**104.5**

OPTION NINE

¼ c. oatmeal	2.5	13	1.5	75.5
½ tbsp. peanut butter	2	1.5	4	50
Totals	**4.5**	**14.5**	**5.5**	**125.5**

OPTION TEN

	Protein	Carbs	Fat	Calories
¼ c. high-fiber cereal	3	11	1	65
¼ c. skim milk	2	3	0	20
Total	**5**	**14**	**1**	**85**

REPLENISH MEALS

Men

Goal:	Protein 5-10	Carbs 20-25	Fat 0-5	Calories 100-185
OPTION ONE				
1 slice whole-grain bread	3	14	2	86
½ tbsp. peanut butter	2	1.5	4	50
Total	**5**	**15.5**	**6**	**136**
OPTION TWO				
2 flavored rice cakes	2	22	0	96
¼ c. fat-free cottage cheese	7	2.5	0	38
Total	**9**	**24.5**	**0**	**134**
OPTION THREE				
½ c. low-fat yogurt	7	20	0	108
Total	**7**	**20**	**0**	**108**
OPTION FOUR				
1 light English muffin	5	23	1	121
Total	**5**	**23**	**1**	**121**
OPTION FIVE				
Small granola bar	2	15	3	95
⅓ c. plain Greek yogurt	8	3	0	44
¼ c. blueberries	0	4	0	16
Total	**10**	**22**	**3**	**155**

OPTION SIX

1 serving baked chips	2	21	3	119
½ oz. beef jerky	7	1	1	41
Total	**9**	**22**	**4**	**160**

OPTION SEVEN

1 apple	1	22	0	92
1 piece string cheese	5	0	2	38
Total	**6**	**22**	**2**	**130**

OPTION EIGHT

1 serving pretzels	2	21	0	92
½ tbsp. peanut butter	2	1.5	4	50
Totals	**4**	**22.5**	**4**	**142**

OPTION NINE

½ banana	0	15	0	64
¼ c. low-fat cottage cheese	7	3	2.5	62.5
Totals	**7**	**18**	**2.5**	**126.5**

OPTION TEN

Energy bar	5	24	2	134
Total	**5**	**24**	**2**	**134**

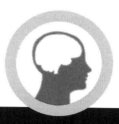

SECTION 3:
Mental Edge

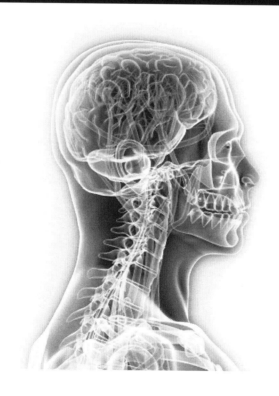

CHAPTER TEN

Eliminating Barriers

Emotional Eating

Research demonstrates the importance of matching a diet to the individual due to genetic uniqueness. The obesity epidemic has prompted the need for better understanding of the aspects necessary for permanent weight loss, but research consistently shows a lack of focus on the psychological components of eating. Most of us can admit to a desire to change certain areas of our bodies, but if holistic self-improvement is the goal, identification of behaviors that could stand a tune-up as well, are also necessary. Unfortunately, rather than embracing a problem-solving and solution-focused approach, many individuals replace positive actions with self-criticism. As unintentional as it may be, it can manifest in unhealthy eating behaviors, such as severe dietary restriction, emotional eating, and even binge eating. Whether it is unacknowledged fear or other disquieting emotions managed poorly, or it is prompted by unrealistic dietary restraint or rigid food rules, health and wellness goals often remain elusive as a result of these behaviors. The psychology of eating is foundational. It must be addressed if one is to realize the goals of comprehensive and sustainable weight loss.

Dietary restraint can create significant physiological hunger. Variables including specific portion sizes, rigid meal times, particular foods and combinations of foods being avoided, and inflexible eating guidelines that can lead to such severe and uncomfortable hunger, build an environment that makes binge eating seem almost inevitable. Obese individuals who binge eat "are likely to choose rigid diets and have little tolerance for deviations from the diet" (Head, 2002, p. 24). Rigidity solicits both physiological and psychological consequences including hunger and emotional discomfort. For example, dieters often express feelings of being out of control. You may relate to the "I was good for a few days, but then I fell off the wagon" effect. The likelihood and severity of binge eating, as well as the factors related to weight loss sustainability, are obviously influenced heavily by psychology, in essence, how we think, which directly impacts how we feel, and finally, how we act. To understand how these factors relate to us, we have to be willing to go to some uncomfortable places. It isn't necessary that we like it, but we need to practice seeing the value in it.

Psyched UP!

Eating behaviors are impacted by "psychological factors such as anxiety, mood, perfectionism, emotion dysregulation, disturbed body image and self-esteem" (Hewitt & Flett, 1991; Sassaroli & Ruggiero, 2005; Markey & Vander Wal; Costarelli, Demerzi, & Stamou, 2009, p. 240). Difficulties in identifying and managing emotions impact food behaviors as well. When one is unskilled at identifying emotions, use of destructive coping methods for emotional management increases. Lacking the ability to know what one is feeling transcends toward a "problem orientation" mindset and can lead to actions being taken with the intention of avoiding or reducing aversive feelings. A number of potentially negative psychological implications, all increasing in severity, have been associated with a problem orientation including anxiety, neuroticism, hopelessness, depression, suicidal ideation, and health complaints.

> Emotional eating is not about food errors—it is about thinking errors.

Emotional Eating— It's Not About Food

The vast majority of individuals who struggle with some form of dysfunctional eating have dieted in the past. The emphasis placed on food and weight, coupled with stringent and unrealistic dietary management practices, sets one up for a chaotic relationship with food. Studies show the strong tendency of dieters, when compared to non-dieters, to overeat, even after having a large meal. Counterregulatory eating, what researchers call the "What the Hell Effect," is a phenomenon that might resonate with you.

Recall the last time you felt guilty about a poor food decision. Perhaps you ate two slices of pizza at a party and you had committed to just one. Next thing you know, you've devoured the mini cheesecakes on the dessert table. Did the thought, "Well, I already screwed up, so I might as well…" cross your mind? Scientists have replicated this behavior in the lab. They brought in a group of people who were hungry and had not had a meal in a few hours. One third of the group were given a small milkshake to tide them over; another third drank two rather large milkshakes that would leave anyone feeling pretty darn full; and the other third got nothing and were told they were just going to be food tasters. All the groups were then separated, and each person was individually asked to rate a different variety of snacks. They were provided with various bowls of cookies and crackers and given permission to eat freely. Care to guess what the researchers found?

The non-dieters in the group who had downed the two large shakes tasted the snacks and rated them quickly, barely having any extra; the one-shake group had a bit more to eat while rating; the hungry group finished off the snacks. Not surprising. The dieters, however, demonstrated the opposite. Those who had two shakes ate more snacks than the other two groups. "Might as well..." right?

Do you see how this thinking is faulty? Emotional eating is not about food errors—it is about thinking errors.

Emotional eating is also a symptom of feeling errors. Feelings are not inherently "bad," but the way in which we interpret them can lead to negative outcomes. Among my clients, stress and anxiety are the most common emotions to precede emotional eating. Without a thought, they will say their hands are in the junk food. The automatic nature of this behavior requires an intentional reinterpretation of the feeling if the goal is to respond differently. For example, you might hear yourself say, "I'm so stressed!" In turn, this thought could morph into "I'll never get this done on time!" The second thought can prompt even greater anxiety, thus perpetuating the cycle. To interrupt the cycle, you must be able to notice the error first, and then respond with objectivity.

These thinking errors are common with addicts of any sort. Cognitive distortions aren't necessarily based in reality, but served a protective role at some point. Unfortunately, they often lead to faulty beliefs, misinterpreted feelings and subsequently, harmful actions. Emotional eating is, in essence, an ineffective coping mechanism designed to protect the individual from an emotion. The problem is that following the eating, the emotion

> Feelings are not inherently "bad," but the way in which we interpret them can lead to negative outcomes.

still exists. Would it not be more effective to learn how to manage the emotion as opposed to running from it?

Acknowledging Our Errors

Ignoring the consequences and implications of our actions may seem easier than acknowledging them sometimes. Years of struggle seem to lead toward either the adoption of a fatalistic, victimhood mentality or a galvanized commitment to exposure and vulnerability. This willingness to accept one's self "as is," is necessary for change to occur. Change can be scary, it can be difficult, and it takes constant vigilance and intentional effort. It's often uncomfortable, but it's worth it. Justifying our actions—or inaction—relieves us of fear we might suffer regarding the time, effort, or possible setbacks that change involves, but only temporarily. When faced repeatedly with the question of whether or not to change, isn't the question itself a good enough indicator that change is due?

The individual who says, "If I hit 200 pounds, then I'll know something needs to be done" or "I'll start Monday" may never take action unless the change is defined as necessary, realistic, and meaningful. I have seen many a Monday turn into the next Monday, into the next Monday, and so forth.

Tune in to your food frequency. Emotional eating is not about food. We can often get in our own way through faulty logic, which leads to eating outside of hunger. Ask yourself honestly what you want to accomplish. Write it out. Make a list of the areas of your life you would like to change and get specific about how your life would be different as a result. Refer to Appendix A for Quick Recovery from Setbacks Activity.

Eliminating Barriers

- Fear attached to a goal can stop you dead in your tracks and is often related to self beliefs. You can attach to it or match it with courage and forge ahead.

- You feel what your mind believes. What if you believed that the feeling you've named "fear" is actually excitement of a future possibility?

- How might you act if you said, "I'm excited about this!" rather than, "I'm worried I can't do it"? Would your behavior change?

CHAPTER ELEVEN

Utilizing Our Internal Voices

All of us have felt conflicted—pulled in different directions simultaneously. The internal forces pushing us toward a certain path can be difficult to understand, and competing interests can leave us feeling mentally chaotic. More often than not, this psychological tug-of-war is the result of emotion—the push-pull between our values and the meaning we've attached to them.

We are products of our experiences. When we're acting with intention, we notice our choices and the opportunities to make them with more clarity. However, if we do not take the time to recognize them, the opposing voices inside of us can drain us of energy and lead to confusion.

> We are products of our experiences.

The voices vie for equal airtime. One may shout, "You can do this!" while the other might be resoundingly fierce in its condemnation of your motivation. "Just give up," it says. "What makes you think this time will be any different?"

An old Cherokee Indian tale demonstrates this concept well.

A Cherokee is telling his grandson about a fight that is going on inside himself. He said it is between two wolves.

One is evil: anger, envy, sorrow, regret, fearful thinking, greed, arrogance, self-pity, guilt, resentment, inferiority, lies, false pride, superiority, and ego.

The other is good: joy, peace, love, hope, serenity, humility, kindness, benevolence, empathy, generosity, truth, compassion, and faith.

The grandson thought about it for a minute and then asked his grandfather, "Which wolf wins?"

The Cherokee simply replied, "The one I feed."

The tale demonstrates the importance of personal responsibility. In everything, we have a choice. The difference between the individual who succumbs to lostness and complacency, however, and the person who can tune in to the challenge of an endeavor with zest and fortitude is attentional awareness. When we take responsibility for

> In everything, we have a choice.

recognizing, assessing, and cultivating choices in life, opportunities are created for personal growth and enjoyment.

The wolf inside of us that bares its teeth in rebellion against personal growth is one that can be tamed. It will always be there, but we decide whether it's growling negativity will be fed.

Recognition—The First Step Toward Emotional Intelligence

Clients come to see me knowing they need to do something different, but their stories vary significantly. Some are older athletes who were once stars of their college sport teams but have left their once-active lives behind. Others have always battled their weight, describing memories as salient as if they happened yesterday of being taunted by schoolmates. Most freely admit how they've harmed their bodies and watched the weight pile on over the years. Many express disappointment and regret for not choosing to intervene sooner. But not surprisingly, most rarely understand their actions.

The "why" questions abound. "Why did I just keep ignoring the aches and pains, the number on the scale, and the heaving breathing!" If they knew the answers, would they know how to change? If I told them, "You say you want one thing but your actions aren't in line with your desires," could they identify the next step to take toward a new way of living?

Most can't. They want to change, but they don't know how.

Recognizing the mind's occurrences is one of the first steps toward mastering the awareness necessary for cultivating the self-understanding these individuals desire. The mindsets with which they approach their circumstances are largely dependent upon their attitudes—what they choose to pay attention to and how they perceive it. Your approach not only influences your psyche, but your body as well.

Some believe they have it figured out. "I just need tools to use when I want to eat," they say in frustration.

One couple came in together seeking support in changing the wife's behavior. "She snacks at night," the husband explained. "When we're in separate rooms watching TV, I can hear her go into the kitchen and go through the cupboards. She knows what she's doing. She's not even hungry! It's a mindset, and she doesn't have it!"

> Your approach not only influences your psyche, but your body as well.

The wife looked at me helplessly. "I know what to do! I just don't do it. I don't know how to stop it!" she said.

The language we use is telling. She describes her struggle as if there is a demon inside her, pulling the strings, clawed hands on the gears which guide her thoughts and actions. She wants the demon gone, yet she continues to feed it. But what is she really feeding?

I could tell her to go for a walk when she wants to eat, call a friend, or play a video game with her son, and any of these activities might serve a temporarily successful role in distracting her. But would it not make more sense to break the surface to learn about what is eating her up inside, and work toward a deeper understanding rather than trying the same thing repeatedly and remaining static in her efforts?

The majority of clients want a quick fix. Immediate gratification—the "give me something now so I can feel better" mentality—is a major reason why individuals cannot keep their weight off. Many people are too impatient and unwilling to do the work to reap the more permanent rewards, believing that alternative behaviors will solve their problems. They are necessary; however, they are also temporary. Without focusing on the reasons and incentives for behavior, we miss identifying their staying power.

> Without focusing on the reasons and incentives for behavior, we miss identifying their staying power.

Emotional Intelligence

Over dinner one evening I caught up with a friend who was soon to have surgery for a neck injury. Unable to lift weights over the last few weeks, her injury was serious enough that the doctor wanted to operate as quickly as possible. As upset as I knew she was about her situation, she spoke to me about a friend whom she'd recently chatted with online.

She updated him about her condition and complained about how annoyed she was regarding her lack of activity. She looked up at me with tear-filled eyes and said, "He told me that he has brain cancer and only has six months to live...." Her voice trailed off briefly. "Whether big or small, we're all suffering. It made me take stock. I felt awful having complained about my stuff after hearing what he was going through."

"It's all relative," I replied. "We're involved in our own lives and we get caught up in our own pain. It's completely normal for you to be upset about your situation, but you get to choose whether you stay locked in the mires of negativity and continue wallowing in self-pity, or 'take stock' like you said and focus on what you are *able* to do. You've got choices."

Choices inherently dictate a focus on personal responsibility. We continue coming back to this concept for good reason. Many individuals get in their own way by perceiving a lack of choices or automatically viewing the situation as black and white. Our perceptions are influenced by the beliefs we hold about ourselves,

> Choices inherently dictate a focus on personal responsibility.

and subsequently, impact our decisions. Choices are the spaces between the events in our lives and our responses, but recognizing them requires a pause.

Attention.

Attunement.

We have to be deliberate if we want to notice the space and use it. We must intentionally slow down long enough to think.

Our beliefs often undermine our value and lead to outcomes that do not serve our best interests. The ability to accurately assess our circumstances, particularly within the emotional realm, is called emotional intelligence (EI). It is developed through improvements in both the cognitive and behavioral dimensions of attitude, values development, and resilience, and is used frequently in the treatment of compulsive eating.

Emotional intelligence requires practice tuning in to the emotional signals of the body and the thought processes accompanying them. Recall the

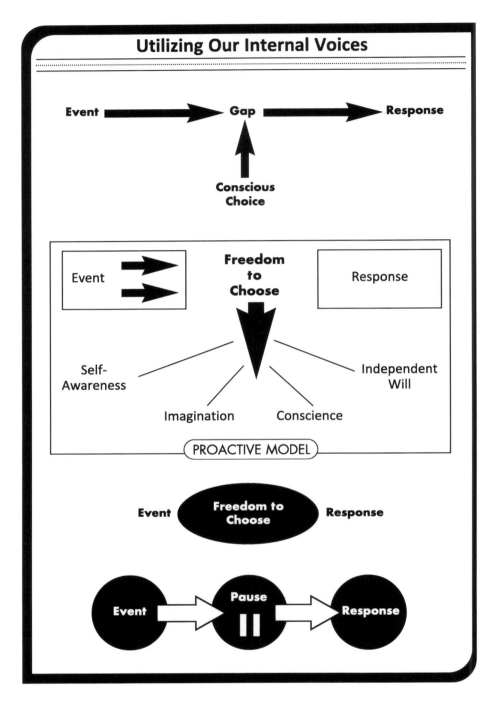

alternative behaviors we discussed? Practicing mind-body awareness means you will learn how to know when to use them! EI can mean the difference between adopting new habits with openness even in the face of difficulty or allowing discouragement to cause abandonment of a goal.

Low emotional intelligence can manifest in impulsive behaviors like emotional eating. Emotional eating is akin to hitting the snooze button when the alarm goes off. Like the alarm, our emotions are

> We must intentionally slow down long enough to think.

cues to pay attention. "Wake up!" Without EI, these cues are missed, or in this context, actively avoided. A person may discern discomfort, but not pause to assess the feeling. Instead food is used, but it delays the inevitable. Just like you have to eventually wake up from slumber, after a binge the emotions that prompted the eating are right there waiting.

Imagine the alternative—developing the ability to effectively notice, accurately assess, and

> Emotional eating is akin to hitting the snooze button when the alarm goes off.

non-judgmentally acknowledge your emotions. With higher-level emotional functioning comes enhanced cognitive flexibility. Individuals who lack these skills tend to spend much of their lives in a position of avoidance, missing out on valuable experiences and reprogramming their internal alarm clocks to a less reliable and accurate frequency. This avoidance behavior is common among those unable to maintain weight loss. Greater flexibility in thought response has been shown to be key to weight-loss permanence.

Food is the medium used in compulsive eating to avoid or relieve anxiety or discomfort. Consider the individual who is experiencing an acutely stressful situation and drives through the nearest Dairy Queen. He may recognize that he is not hungry but eats to temporarily alleviate his anxiety and replace it with short-term pleasure.

A client's email to me demonstrates this well. "I had a disturbing conversation with my brother last night," he said. "When I got off the phone I wanted sugar. I needed sugar!"

I hear sentiments like this repeatedly. We value having answers. We like to feel sure. We're not so great with uncertainty. The unknowns of life can lead to discomfort, and under circumstances that feel out of our control, eating may be used as a measure to regain it. However, research indicates that lasting mood changes are not accomplished with eating. Using a modified "mood-freezing manipulation" technique, researchers have shown even when coupled with the belief that the mood could be changed, compulsive eating results in transient, temporarily uplifting emotion. Often, the binge produces higher levels of negative emotion as a tremendous amount of guilt is experienced for indulging, accompanied by further loss of control. Emotional intelligence skills alleviate the need for food to be used as an emotion regulation tool, and among binge eaters, creates a stronger likelihood for dieting success and weight loss sustainability.

> Greater flexibility in thought response has been shown to be key to weight-loss permanence.

Developing Awareness

I have a tendency to hang onto things. Maybe you can relate. My old running shoes that carried me over the finish line with a personal best time last year sit quietly in my closet, the cushioning and support system completely broken down. The sweatshirt I acquired over a decade ago during college, which I never wear, takes up space in my dresser. It leaves no room for the

> " Emotional distress that is markedly high in arousal will often cause one to fail in thinking through the consequences of a behavior, leading to self-defeating actions.

newer, more sophisticated clothing I've purchased. I know I don't need them. They aren't practical. They're producing clutter. Yet I refuse to let them go.

On a more life-altering, but less tangible level, as I write this I'm acutely aware of my concern about defining how and who I will be without the active pursuit of physique competition. I've come to a point in my career and life where my desire and intentions for competing have changed in a way that leaves me dissatisfied and questioning what it would look like to continue. And yet, almost out of obligation, I feel a need to choose another competition and plan my attack. Shoes are one thing, but life goals are another.

When I moved into my new home I became aware of the "stuff" I had accumulated over the years. I was reminded again of lingering, far-from-useful stuff when my mom came to visit recently. Yes, there is tangible stuff and metaphorical, psychological stuff. You've probably referred to this stuff as baggage. Our baggage can create barriers in our ability to achieve goals and realize our potential, but we're often not even aware of what's in our suitcases.

From birth, we begin to develop a sense of what is important. Through our interactions, and lack thereof, we attach meanings to experience. Our worldviews take shape and we develop beliefs about who we want to be and who we are.

Life hands us stuff that we collect and categorize into personal beliefs, values, attitudes, thoughts, emotions, coping skills, and patterns of behavior. Experiences create scripts that etch themselves into our brains. Often, our collections are hidden away, collecting dust, until certain events initiate a download. It's not necessarily intentional. It's survival.

"I'm so angry! I just want to hit something!" my client screamed.

She hunched her shoulders up as she attempted to prevent the flood gates from breaking wide open. Proving too strong to avoid, her emotions came gushing down her cheeks.

"I don't know what to do!" she sobbed. "I want to run away! When I was a child I would run to the forest. I had a spot where I'd just sit by myself. When I got older I started using drugs, and I smoked all the time. Last night I smoked three cigarettes. I can't believe I did that. I haven't smoked in fifteen years!"

Her choking sobs and labored breathing continued as I slowly reached over and handed her a box of tissue. I said to her softly, "You did what you did because you wanted to feel better. There was a reason for it, and it used to work, but now your old stuff doesn't take away your pain so well."

Behaviors that effectively reduced her pain, confusion, or hurt in the past didn't mature with her. As a child, she could use them without discomfort. Now they were undermining her growth. It was time to expose the roots of her reliance on them and begin developing more appropriate coping skills.

In the throes of emotion, the use of our old stuff may not be so apparent. A binge eater may realize halfway into a binge, or even following the binge, that she relied on an old behavior to "remedy" a negative emotion or to forget a painful memory. Dieters, for example, may ordinarily be able to fight the temptation of a decadent dessert or rich foods to pursue the long-term goals of a leaner body and good health. When emotionally upset, however, the importance of the long-term goals fades in comparison to the urgent need to feel better.

Emotional distress that is markedly high in arousal will often cause one to fail in thinking through the consequences of a behavior, leading to self-defeating actions. This confirms the need for skill development in emotional recognition and reasoning. We will always experience feelings! The manner in which we respond to them will move us closer to or further from our goals.

Take, for example, the husband who doesn't want to confront his wife about his disappointment regarding a situation in their marriage. Instead, he retreats to his office. He has learned it is better to keep quiet. Watching his father get screamed at and reprimanded by his mother when he'd approach her with his feelings was incentive enough to avoid conflict. When he was upset with his mom as a child he'd disappear and distract himself with his GI Joes. Now, however, his avoidance creates hurt and confusion. His old stuff is ineffective and damaging.

For my client it wasn't okay to feel. Having suffered through significant emotional and physical abuse as a child, she learned to survive by shutting off her feelings. As she learns to trust that they are now safe to experience, she feels uncomfortable and foreign in her body. Overweight and unhappy, she spent years stuffing her emotions down deep with food.

Psyched UP!

Dieting success and compulsive eating are clearly related to emotion regulation. As psychological discomfort increases, the use of negative coping behaviors rises in order to relieve or avoid the perceived unpleasant feeling. Described as causing a breakdown in one's impulse control, emotional distress, as explained in some theories, "impairs one's motivation or one's ability to exert self-control, and some postulate self-destructive intentions arising from the [negative] moods" (Tice et al., p. 53). For example, excessive eating increases among overweight people when they are anxious or depressed. In addition, induction of anxiety among obese individuals and a bad mood in dieters has been shown to cause increases in food consumption. Like a negative feedback loop, eating increases with negative emotion, which triggers more eating, and as the person ruminates on the breakdown of his or her dietary constraints, an escalation of distress results.

> Assessment, decluttering, organization, and identification serves to create awareness of the behaviors worth staying attached to, as well as those better replaced.

Old stuff likes to hang on. When we are feeling weak, tired, and with diminished resolve, we revert to the old stuff more easily. Despite our awareness of its consequences, the old stuff doesn't just disappear. Changing it takes a careful, well-executed plan. Like a bone marrow transplant, you must clean out what is there first.

Lasting change requires closure of the old to bring in the new. Assessment, decluttering, organization, and identification serves to create awareness of the behaviors worth staying attached to, as well as those better replaced. This work is a necessary and integral part of developing the mindset necessary for bolstering the commitment it will take to achieve your goals.

Piece of Mind

- When we're acting with intention, we notice our choices and the opportunities to make decisions with more clarity.
- Attentional awareness is taking responsibility for recognizing, assessing, and cultivating choices in life, which in turn creates opportunities for personal growth and enjoyment.
- Your mindset is largely dependent upon your attitude and influences how you will approach situations. Your attitude dictates what you choose to pay attention to and how you perceive it.
- Immediate gratification—as a result of low self-regulation skills—is a primary factor in poor weight-loss maintenance.
- The need for skill development in emotional recognition and reasoning is great. Emotional intelligence gives you the ability to think through consequences and avoid self-defeating actions.

CHAPTER TWELVE

Moving From Motivation to Commitment

CLIENTS EXPRESS a strong desire to change their eating habits and fitness levels the first time we meet. Some are fed up with being overweight, lethargic, and unable to fit into their clothes. Others are facing a serious medical crisis. On the opposite end of the continuum are fitness fanatics who are striving for the upper echelon in athletics, physique, or other competitive endeavors. The first two groups often require a shift in thinking.

As we begin the change process, I'm met with a furrowed brow, a frown, and a concerned and somewhat dumbfounded, "Hmmmm," when I explain the behaviors and mindset associated with permanent success. While the thought of change may initially be scary, we have all experienced success and can relate back to the effort it required to achieve it. We made decisions and possibly sought guidance in doing so, and we attempted to behave or think differently.

When I realized, for example, that I would get nothing accomplished by studying in my dorm room, I found a spot on the top floor of the library and would study there for hours. My thoughts went from frustrated musings of killing my roommate for having her music blaring to thinking, *I've got to make this happen. Find a place to get it done!*

You are reading this book, ideally with thoughts resembling, *I'm really going to do it this time—it's do or die!* You may not know the precise outcomes of what you are about to engage in, but the process will show you where your hidden potential resides. If you are out of your comfort zone, that's right where you're supposed to be.

This concept of process awareness separates those individuals who set goals but "just can't seem to get the job done" from those who take the bull by the horns, do whatever it takes, and exhibit the strength of mind, drive, and determination to let not a single thing get in their way. This is the difference between motivation and commitment.

I've been in both positions and in between at various points in my life. I attended a concert and was fortunate enough to speak with the lead singer of the band. After that

> If you are out of your comfort zone, that's right where you're supposed to be.

evening I was hell-bent on auditioning for *X-Factor* and learning to play the guitar. Without an audition to speak of, my untouched guitar now stands lonely in a far corner of my living room. Boy was I motivated! I have given up on other endeavors too. Does this mean I am unsuccessful, lazy, or a failure? More often than not, I pursue new things with an almost rabid obsession. Those that stick are the ones to which I was committed. You can assess the difference by asking yourself some key questions and taking a personal assessment. The following questions are often helpful in providing you with greater perspective:

Why is this important to me?

How will it make a difference in my life?

What are the incentives in doing the work it will take to accomplish?

Is the goal one I can view as a challenge rather than a burden?

What are the costs versus the benefits?

Is now the time for this? If not now, when?

The areas of your life that you will not give up on, no matter what, are linked by one thing—commitment.

Motivation operates on a continuum. It waxes and wanes. Mood states, emotions, and the situation can influence motivation levels. For example, John who has lost fifty pounds, is exercising regularly and contacts me daily with questions. He returns home from a long and tiring day of work and thinks, "I'd really like to just order a pizza for dinner." He heads into his kitchen, however, to prepare a healthy burrito with his whole-grain tortilla, chicken breast, low-fat cheese, and veggies. Was he motivated? Not exactly. He wanted pizza—to have his dinner cooked for him. Despite his situational fatigue he made a positive decision. How did John bypass the urge to order pizza? The answer lies in the components of commitment.

Recalibrating Your Mental Set Point

You now understand how motivation is influenced by a mood—a feeling—and how it can change rapidly. Commitment, on the other hand, is much less dictated by emotion or circumstance. It's the action of "just doing it," even if it's not your first impulse. At the commitment level, your mental set point has been recalibrated. Those who succeed are those who are committed to challenging themselves. They capitalize on their strengths and objectively assess their weaknesses. This objectivity allows for a focus on the facts. It is evidence-based. If you can approach your situation in this manner, you will more easily take responsibility for your behavior and see failures as opportunities for growth and new understanding. You will find that you wallow less in the midst of a "bad day" or a negative circumstance. All of us have felt fatigued, felt like tapping out, or have questioned how much longer we could persevere. Yet we've kept going. This is commitment.

One of my clients said it best with this comment: "Once I get this new job, get some normalcy back into my life and start getting back into working out, hopefully things will get back on track. I would really like to lose another eight- to ten-pounds but I just don't know if it will happen if I don't work

Motivation	Commitment
The goal changes with mood	The goal is static and enduring
Altered by physical and emotional status	Driven by objectivity
Perceived to be related to education and knowledge	Colored by a future orientation
Driven by impulses and drives	Embodies skill in emotion regulation
	Delayed gratification

> The areas of your life that you will not give up on, no matter what, are linked by one thing—commitment.

harder. I can say that now but doing it is another thing. Like I knew that I should've worked out tonight but instead I just came home and played with my son. My motivation has so much of a swing to it. One day I'm motivated, and one day I'm not. I really have to push myself some days."

The committed individual recognizes that this is part of the game—expects it even. There will be ups, there will be downs, and there will be situations that are not ideal. But the committed person operates with a sense of mastery and purpose.

"Hopefully" is not a part of their vocabulary.

Motivation to change occurs in stages: you may be interested, for example, in learning about permanent weight loss but not yet ready to engage in the intentional behaviors it will require. Even so, if you are deliberately seeking information to increase your awareness and knowledge of the topic you are exhibiting self-efficacy. One who believes in their personal influence of a situation and takes responsibility demonstrates high self-efficacy. The greater the belief in one's intrinsic ability to succeed and achieve an outcome, the less the difficult circumstances will be viewed as insurmountable. Take a moment to assess how quickly you give up when working toward a goal. How often do you hear yourself say, "I should," but you do not follow through? Refer to Appendix B for the Motivation vs. Commitment Activity.

Piece of Mind

- Change requires intentional, purposeful, and deliberate behavior and thinking.

- Present-moment awareness supports recognition of current behavior, cognition, and emotion so that new, more effective, goal-congruent replacements may be made.

CHAPTER THIRTEEN

Taking Risks: Developing a Growth Mindset

RELOCATING across the country to create the Mental Edge program as the Wellness Director for The Diet Doc was one of the most life-altering decisions I've made to date. Yet, it took me a matter of seconds to begin planning to move. Risky? Absolutely.

When I was a kindergartner, my mom debated holding me back a year because I was so shy. In grade school I was scared to walk up to the Taco Bell counter to ask for a napkin. It wasn't until my teens and early college years that I began taking risks, eager to see what opportunities were ahead of me. I moved toward challenges that required me to stretch, my love of learning nurtured on the outskirts of my comfort zone.

Our mindsets help explain the reasons for our behavior. Each of us varies in our abilities and the choices we make to either be active participants in our lives or victims of circumstance. Many miss out on the richness of life's experiences because of fear, learned helplessness, or distortions in thinking. Additionally, our worldviews and personal beliefs can lead to a tendency to stay engaged in very "safe" activities. Afraid of making mistakes, we may seek endeavors perceived to guarantee success. We desire the outcome—the end result—often forgetting the value of the road we must travel to get there. Dieters can demonstrate this mentality. Desperate to lose the excess weight, they jump on faddish, cookie-cutter, quick-fix approaches that promise quick results. The reasons for their decisions are many; however, a common theme emerges consistently during my interviews with potential clients: low self-confidence combined with unrealistic expectations. My goal is not only to guide these individuals toward weight loss, but to teach them how to begin trusting themselves through the process. I want them to learn to thrive on challenge and to see each new experience as a door opening to possibility. Through this work, they learn to love learning, and although they may not like making mistakes, they don't measure their worth by those failures.

Dr. Carol Dweck, leading behavioral researcher at Stanford University, describes two mindsets that individuals tend to move toward: fixed versus growth. She has conducted research on children to determine how various models

> Many miss out on the richness of life's experiences because of fear, learned helplessness, or distortions in thinking.

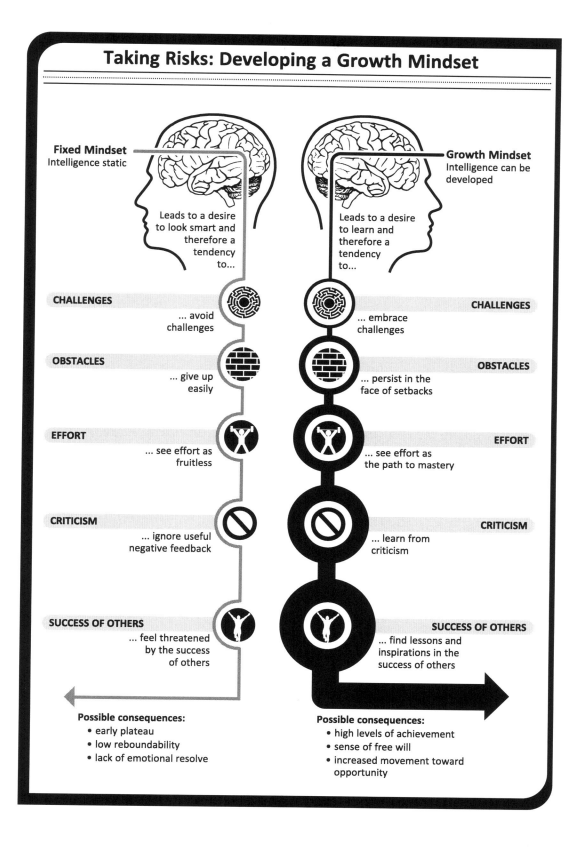

> "Your perception of your ability to succeed will determine what you choose to engage in, how much effort you'll make before giving up, and your assessment of stress.

of intelligence impact achievement. These models, the entity model and incremental model, demonstrate varying beliefs regarding whether intelligence is a relatively "fixed" entity or more malleable and can be developed incrementally. Dr. Dweck found that the junior-high-school students who attributed their success to effort and who believed that intelligence could be developed through learning, more effectively achieved their educational goals. When setbacks were encountered, these students, when compared with those who believed their intelligence was "fixed," attributed the mistakes less to their personal abilities and exhibited an increase in effort as opposed to demonstrating helplessness. Two years later when these same groups of students were compared on scores of mathematics achievement, those who believed that intelligence could be learned were outperforming the others and demonstrated significantly higher levels of motivation.

Dweck's theory sounds similar to Bandura's concept of self-efficacy, which describes the belief in one's ability to influence the events in life despite the possibility of setbacks or unpredictable occurrences. One with high self-efficacy would exhibit a growth mindset. What does this mean for you? Your perception of your ability to succeed will determine what you choose to engage in, how much effort you'll make before giving up,

and your assessment of stress. We are not solely fixed or growth-minded, however. A growth mindset can be achieved with practice. I call the movement from a fixed to a growth mindset, attitudinal positioning. If you imagine mindset on a continuum, you can position your attitude and perception anywhere between the two ends.

Recall fat loss being a positional phenomenon. Once you get a taste for the success you can experience as you ride along the continuum, your commitment to residing there strengthens. With every incremental movement downward on the scale, your self-control is fortified. The concept translates to attitude as well.

Practiced, positive perception begets a reinforcement of will. I notice immediately when my attitude slides backward, and I am quick to flip the switch.

You possess the power to become who you want to be. First, however, comes learning how to be present-minded in order to assess your current situations. In other

> You possess the power to become who you want to be."

words, you must develop a new level of awareness. Living on auto-pilot is no longer an option if you wish to view your life in 360 degrees, make wiser decisions, and manage your life more effectively.

No blinders.

No hiding.

Look at this new awareness as mindfulness, giving you the freedom to move with purpose toward developing a plan for change. Rather than reacting and moving in a fixed manner, a present-focused approach allows for a repositioning of your attitudes for stretching, digging, engaging, learning, and growing.

It is dynamic and fluid.

Mindfulness is perspective-taking illuminated. Goals of value take on greater meaning in this context, and those deemed just slightly important can be reevaluated. Important to consider, however, is that despite a goal's meaning, it many never come to fruition due to inadequate planning. Few take the time to assess or anticipate potential barriers, the mind being one of the most influential.

What's the Plan, Man?

Imagine leaving on a 1,000-mile road trip without having checked the air pressure of your spare tire. One roadblock that most do not consider is the mind. Let's assess the hurdles it can present. Assuming that either the tire is filled adequately or just forgetting completely to check it, you set off down the highway. Your gas tank is full, you've got some snacks to hold you until lunch time, and you compiled a playlist for your journey. *I'm such a good planner*, you think to yourself. Suddenly you feel a jolt, there is an audible thud, and then you smell burning rubber. Your heart's beating rapidly as you guide the car slowly to the shoulder. Getting out carefully to inspect the situation, you see that the rear driver's-side tire is deflated. Grumbling as you open the trunk to retrieve your spare and jack, you berate yourself for not securing the AAA program you received in the mail recently. You lift the floor board and immediately your stomach is in your throat. Where is the tire?

Planning is imperative for any important goal and part of smart planning is asking the question, "What could go wrong?" Researchers call this *defensive pessimism*, and it's a skill many of us lack. Learning to anticipate what might occur gives us the ability to plan ahead. One of the most effective ways of answering this question is to identify what the barriers have been in the past. Take a moment now to assess your previous setbacks. Now you have a starting point from which to begin planning a different approach. Refer to Appendix C1 for Developing a Plan for Hunger and Cravings Activity.

> Planning is imperative for any important goal and part of smart planning is asking the question, "What could go wrong?"

The Mind's Roadblocks

Learning to be mindful does not necessarily mean we will prevent roadblocks from occurring every time. There are many things, especially environmentally, that are out of our control. But it does mean that we will be able to view them more objectively when they do occur. Sometimes in this process we realize our choices have not been ours. Allow me to explain.

My new 400-pound client walked through the doors of The Diet Doc. I knew nothing about him. He timidly removed his coat, and barely breathing, took a place in the chair closest to the door. This is typical of most people I see. Should they perceive the need to escape, a sprint across five feet of office space is not required. I joke, but this behavior is telling. Escape artists are what many of my obese or overweight clients have become. Adept at avoiding what they do not want to see, hear, or feel, they have insulated themselves from what makes them most human. The moment this burly man sat down, his eyes welled up with tears.

Squinting with discomfort, he explained that he had struggled with being fat his entire life. His parents divorced when he was in sixth grade in a brutally ambivalent and conflict-filled fanfare of events. Living with his mother, who was patronizing and cold, his needs as a young boy growing up without a father and a positive male influence were danced around with passive-aggressive indifference. Ridicule and teasing from his peers at school was a daily occurrence.

"When I'd tell her that I was being teased about my weight," he explained to me, "she'd just say 'ignore it.'"

The message he took from these interactions resulted in a belief that he was unimportant. Speaking up was pointless. When she told him to ignore it, *he* felt ignored. Without the warmth of a growth-minded parent, he had no space to be a boy who was scared, or the room to navigate choices and decisions typical of an eleven-year-old. He could control nothing, despised his mother and yet wanted to love her, was an outcast unworthy of friendship, and bullied by his schoolmates with no recourse.

Except to eat.

Thirty years later he is sitting in my office facing what he doesn't realize are similar circumstances, and he's reacting in the same manner.

Now married with two children he is desperate to provide them with a different experience. He strives to give them some independence and yet provide what he understands to be loving support. His wife has lost a significant amount of weight; however, she has adopted some stringent eating and food rules. Where *his* fear resides in not being able to lose his excess weight and fully participate in his own or his sons' lives, she fears gaining the weight back.

When she sees him eat something she believes to be unhealthy, the attitude begins, the frustrated harrumphs and eye-rolling starts, and you can guess to where this man is transported. He can't make a decision on his own and have it respected, and he can't express himself or it turns aversive and ugly.

Still seeing his mom on a regular basis, he explains how he hates going over to her home.

"My mom is a borderline hoarder. You can't walk through the hallways without knocking something off the walls. Stuff is everywhere. She can't get rid of it. She goes to flea markets and buys stuff thinking that at some point she'll use it. But she doesn't throw other things out. I hate going there. And I get in trouble at home for helping her so much because then I'm neglecting my own home duties."

Again he's in a catch-22. Obligation. In that place there is no room for individual decision-making.

"So how do you handle that? Going there when you don't want to?" I ask.

His eyes glisten again and he says, "I insulate myself from the anger I feel when I go. And a lot of times I just avoid going."

"But you don't and haven't told your mom that you're uncomfortable going or that you don't want to?" I ask, already knowing the answer.

"No. She'd freak out."

Later he speaks of not knowing how to be happy.

"My wife always tells me that I need to do what I know will make me happy, but I don't know what that means."

How can he make choices and try new behaviors if he learned as a young boy that making decisions on his own always resulted in others being upset?

"I drive home from work every night pissed off because I know my wife is going to have the same thing on the table for dinner. I hate having the same thing every single night. She can do that. But I need some variety. Everywhere we go she has to have a cooler packed full of chicken breast or protein bars. Say we're going to a sporting event. I just might want to get a soft pretzel for a meal! If I do, here come the looks, the sighs...."

He tells me about the nights that he'd go through McDonald's and get a Big Mac and super-sized fries for dinner on his way home.

"You eat out of spite sometimes," I said. "It's like you're thinking, 'Fine. You won't let me make my own food decisions around you, or any decisions at all for that matter, I'll show you that I can...and I will.'"

He leaves the trash in the car. Like he wants to be found out.

His mom hoards things. He hoards food. She insulates her life, living in the future, unaware of the present. He insulates his life, living in the past, unaware of how his current decisions are based on past beliefs that are no longer effective. Developing a new attitude—one unencumbered by faulty beliefs and the messages of his childhood—would take time, patience, and practice. The binge eating would need to be anticipated as an automatic reaction to his most common uncomfortable emotions, and he would need to learn to manage his feelings in a more productive, mindful manner.

Piece of Mind

- Greater self-awareness increases authenticity.
- Self check-ins create opportunities to assess thoughts and emotions.
- Practicing awareness facilitates the habit of recognizing personal signs and symptoms of distress and positive emotions.
- Refer to Appendix C2 for the Psychological vs. Physiological Hunger Activity. This activity facilitates skill-building to increase emotional intelligence.

CHAPTER FOURTEEN

Environmental Triggers

THE STOMACH GROWLING often signals normal physiological hunger. If blood sugar has dropped to very low levels, feelings of hypoglycemia such as faintness, headache, and lethargy may occur. These peripheral signals are learned and impact subsequent eating and foraging behaviors. They can be prompted with even a ten percent drop in blood glucose levels. Interestingly, many people rarely experience hunger, often eating in amounts far above what their bodies need! Clearly, for normal and moderate eating to occur, the ability to detect these changes in the body is crucial.

While physiological cues can trigger eating so too can environmental signals. With the increase in external food cues from billboards, radio, and television, for example, more people are eating fast and convenient food, cooking less, and choosing to eat outside of physiological hunger. Termed "food porn," the media's fast food-focused advertising has contributed to the obesity epidemic. On a daily basis, each of us makes an average of 200 food-related decisions. Think back to the discussion on willpower. It is not surprising that an individual would struggle when making changes to eating behavior when being bombarded with messages to "eat, eat, eat!" Interestingly, studies on obese versus normal-weight control subjects indicate higher food-cue responsiveness among the obese. They display greater motivation to consume food, higher sensitivity to food during hunger states, an increased drive toward immediate versus delayed gratification, and increased perception of reward attached to food.

What does this mean? We have our work cut out for us in developing not only the ability to recognize true hunger, but the willingness to take the time to do so. The hypothalamus, the brain's control center, directly impacts memory, learning, emotion, and behavior as related to food and appetite. It acts in tandem with the physiological cues and states that we experience, like hunger and thirst. The learned associations we acquire as a result of pleasurable or aversive eating experiences depend on the hypothalamus as well, and it allows us to make decisions according to environmental stimuli. In essence, your motivations for eating stem largely from your previous experiences operating in conjunction with your surroundings.

> On a daily basis, each of us makes an average of 200 food-related decisions.

Piece of Mind

- There is a reason why we're called creatures of habit. If something feels good, we're more likely to do it again...and again...and again. And this is outside of what we actually choose to learn and "memorize." Our brains release specific hormones related to pleasure and thus create subsequent drives to achieve that same feeling. Before we may even be aware, we're doing something repeatedly.

- Unless the behavior suddenly creates discomfort in our lives, we won't necessarily assess it to be dysfunctional. But like the binge eater, who has "memorized" how to eat in times of stress or anxiety, the guilt; the hiding; or the excessive amounts of money being spent on food, for example, become conscious signals of something "not right."

- Habits are essentially well-worn paths running through our brains. Because habits have become automatic, they are difficult to break. Requiring intense deliberateness and intention, they can be changed, however, and the paths can grow over. New, more effective paths can be carved out.

- The field of neuroplasticity has revealed the brain's amazing capacity to transform itself when stimulated differently and with attention. When working toward habit change, it is important to identify triggers within the environment that can potentially cause breakdowns in self-regulation. Dieters will often express difficulties regarding eating out with friends, smelling certain foods, or passing by their old favorite food establishments. Urges can be intense.

- See Appendix D for the Identifying Barriers to Success activity.

CHAPTER FIFTEEN

Maintenance—Be a Life Athlete!

EVERYTHING UP TO THIS POINT has prepared you for successful maintenance. We created *50 Days to Your Best ~~Body~~ Life* to address the synchronicity between the mind and the body in relation to dieting and sustainable weight loss. There is, in our estimation, no valid reason to move into a goal of weight loss and health without securing the skills that will be necessary to keep the weight off for good. Let's review the key components of weight loss sustainability.

Managing Emotions

The mindset chapters focused on preparing you for a successful dieting experience and included pre-dieting skills and emotional management skills. You are now aware of how imperative effectively coping with emotion is to successful dieting. Not only can emotion lead to mindless and unnecessary eating and subsequent threats to achieving weight loss, individuals who successfully maintain their weight loss demonstrate an ability to monitor and manage internal states more effectively and exhibit behavioral flexibility.

Emotional eating is often prompted by feelings of anxiety or worry, stress, anger, sadness or depression. In an attempt to avoid the feeling, food is used to distract. In a sense, emotional eating is a method of self-protection. Food can provide temporary respite from what has been perceived as negative, however, as we've discussed, the eating typically intensifies the discomfort. Additionally, the ambivalence one experiences can often be a clue to incompatibility between intention and action. Ever been in a situation where you've lied about something and it is "eating you up inside"? That gnawing feeling—that's dissonance. On another level, it is the internal volley you can experience between "knowing what to do" and actually doing it. Specific patterns in thinking, particularly all-or-nothing thinking, catastrophizing, and assumption-making, leave us vulnerable to the vice of emotional eating.

Paying Attention: If you find yourself getting swept away by your emotions and hear statements like "I feel lost" or "I'm so confused," it's time to take a closer look at your emotional management skills. To begin practicing more effective coping, try implementing regularly scheduled self-awareness checks in order to get in touch with your physiological and cognitive states. Assess them as if you were a scientist gathering data.

Just observe. The goal is to become more adept at approaching your circumstances more objectively and nonjudgmentally. Refer to Appendix E1 for the Managing Emotions Activity.

Monitoring Cognitive Distortions

The thinking style common among weight regainers often follows a dichotomous pattern, indicating a lack of flexibility in managing both practical matters or internal/emotional drives and cues. Behavioral flexibility is low among overweight individuals, indicating a more rigid and habitually restrained manner of behaving. Problem-solving skills appear impaired also. This is not surprising in light of the often-subjective nature of emotions. Feelings, when described by most, have meaning attached. A valence. Emotion, after all, is formed based on how we associate with a certain situation.

Becoming a Scientist: To practice a more objective approach, under circumstances in which you feel emotionally vulnerable, you must work toward assessing the situation from a "just the facts" perspective. You can practice this by monitoring your thoughts, assessing the thinking errors you engage in, and then examining your situation in an "evidence-based" manner. Refer to Appendix E2 for the Life Athlete Monitoring Cognitive Distortions Activity.

Implementing Behavioral Flexibility

What might be perceived as counterintuitive to weight loss, behavioral flexibility refers to the ability to respond in a non-rigid manner to varying circumstances. Lower among obese and overweight individuals, it helps to explain their more limited restraint that leads to over-consumption of food in the presence of environmental food cues. Greater restraint and lack of flexibility also leads to counter-regulatory eating, known as the "What the Hell" effect. Recall the previous discussion about a threatening circumstance that lead to overeating and the subsequent thought of "Well, I already screwed up, so I might as well...." The "What the Hell" effect creates disappointment and shame among many dieters.

Break the Ball and Chain: Identify the rules you have put in place for yourself. Assess the previous diets you've engaged in, get a sense for how they have prompted the adoption of behaviors leaving you with a feeling of being tied to a ball and chain. Consider rules that begin with words like "always" or "never." Refer to Appendix E3 for the Life Athlete Implementing Behavioral Flexibility Activity.

Developing Problem-Solving Skills

Among those with limited behavioral flexibility, problem-solving appears to be especially ineffective. Emotional responses to rigid diet rules tend to be more significant and can lead to binge eating and unhealthy compensation. Furthermore, greater discomfort in the presence of hunger is experienced, black and white thinking is engaged in often, stress is often managed by overeating, and emotional eating is common when negative feelings occur. In the context of weight regain, lack of behavioral flexibility can mean a return to baseline habits quickly if these habits are not targeted. Developing more effective problem-solving skills requires practice like the other changes in behavior you are working toward.

Turn On and Tune In: Refer to Appendix E4 for the Life Athlete RADAR Activity to begin implementing the key concepts of problem-solving and self-awareness. Ready? Let's tune your personal RADAR.

Anticipating and Planning Ahead

Individuals who are successful maintainers are adept at recognizing the loop that can occur when emotion is experienced, then food is eaten, which causes additional dissonance and more food consumed, and can intervene earlier in the cycle. They will exhibit more balance by allowing a higher intake at one meal or for a day and either plan to increase activity levels or eat at a more moderate level the next day to compensate. In essence, they demonstrate a more proactive approach to problem-solving and implement a defensively pessimistic stance to stay focused on their goals.

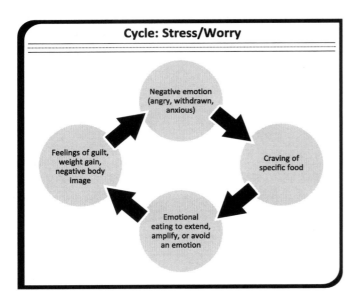

"R" is for Responsibility, Not Restrictions: Overeating often leads to the "What the Hell" effect. Practice a new approach when you have acted in a manner that is creating discomfort. Try saying, "Okay, this is not an ideal situation, but it's also not the end of the world. How can I take responsibility and not beat myself up?" Responsibility-taking doesn't mean saying, "You messed up; it's okay." It also doesn't mean saying, "You messed up; you better not eat anything the rest of the week." Take this a step further and plan for how you can stay true to what is important to you when you're faced with a similar situation in the future. Begin developing a relapse prevention plan by first identifying what your triggers are. Refer to Appendix E5 for the Life Athlete Anticipating and Planning Ahead Activity.

Developing a Proactive Approach to Goal-Striving

"Defensive pessimism" (De Ridder, et al., 2007, p.295) can influence weight regain. Those who have poor emotional intelligence are unable to exhibit the balance necessary to prevent relapses in eating and implement effective coping strategies and stress management practices due to difficulties identifying and managing emotion. The consequences of this lack of skill are numerous and operate on a continuum, but not all hope is lost! Research shows that the event of a threat that has the capacity to create negative emotion may actually be helpful as it can be used as an opportunity for self-regulation.

Two models describe how the factors of self-control and goal-striving operate together to impact self-regulation. These models, in tandem with what the research describes as defensive pessimism, offer new insights into weight maintenance.

In the context of weight maintenance, threats abound that have the capacity to compromise healthy eating, regular exercise, and more importantly, stress management. For example, the goal of establishing new, more effective habits may be negotiated in light of a television advertisement for a pizza or the billboard announcing free ice cream, skipping exercise to attend a dinner out with friends, or choosing to eat the chocolate on a co-worker's desk when stress at work runs high. The limited capacity model asserts that with these accumulating temptations and stressors, the capacity to exert self-control becomes severely limited due to a narrowing of emotional resources, and subsequently, self-regulation falters. In other words, we finally fall apart because we've been working so hard mentally to avoid what we understand won't help us! Like a muscle that fatigues with accumulating work, so too does our self-control.

Strengthening the Muscle of Your Mind: If you are resistance training, you understand and have experienced muscle failure. With progressively heavier loads, the number of reps you can complete decreases. You know you're getting stronger, however, when with the same weight your reps increase. The same holds true with self-control, or what many individuals like to call willpower. Like a muscle, when it is taxed with a challenge, it becomes fatigued. With continued emotional load it would eventually fail, leading to you succumbing to a temptation. With practice, your self-control grows stronger. You can resist temptation with greater ease, and what once felt threatening may not even phase you. Think of something in your life that at one time seemed difficult but is now handled with ease. How did you make the transition? What skills did you implement? Refer to Appendix E6 for the Skills Transfer Activity.

Using Setbacks to Improve Future Behavior

The second model demonstrates the potentially positive impact temptations can impart, bringing the long-term goal to the forefront of the individual's thinking. It emphasizes how frustration, faced when a goal is threatened, can make the goal more prominent. In other words, obstacles can actually create a sense of urgency and prompt a dieter to put forth greater effort. What would this effort look like? Stand by! Imagine yourself assuming a position of power and confidence, behavioral flexibility, anticipation and planning, identification and changing of negative attitudes or cognitions, autonomy and competence, detection and prevention, implementation of objective strategies, and a state of action-preparedness. Did you get that? If not, please re-read. Humor me—this is you as *the Metabolic Inferno!* In essence, everything you've learned from the beginning gels into a cohesive whole so that when you encounter threats to your goal, you can automatically implement your Jedi mind tricks!

It's no wonder, when you consider all the skills that are required for the most powerful mindset, that regainers express a strong sense of perceived effort. How many times have you heard yourself say, "But it's so hard!" The skills listed above are not inherent in one's psychological repertoire and must be learned!

Self-regulation, a big word to explain the strategies one uses when discomfort is experienced, has been the subject of many studies. Researchers have been interested in what happens when individuals experience feelings of stress, and what they've found is that when stress is felt but isn't attached to a specific goal-threat, self-regulatory effort doesn't change; but those who perceive that their goals might be compromised as a result of stress do in fact demonstrate behaviors of planning and damage mitigation. What does this mean? How you *think* about your distress helps to determine its impact on your behavior!

Most importantly, positive efforts were made only when accompanying information existed that conveyed the ability to manage it. For example, support, a plan, or even a mantra developed ahead of time for when difficult situations arise can be crucial. In essence, unrelated to a goal, stress has a tendency to prompt either neutral or negative behaviors that impair goal-striving. When attached to an achievement being worked toward, however, stress in the presence of trust in your personal ability can lead to greater positive effort.

Don't Mistake Frustration for Failure: Think of a person in your life whom you admire. When I do this, I gravitate toward those who are steadfast in their pursuits, who seem never to give up, who are calm under pressure, who demonstrate tenacity and determination, who fall a lot but get right back up, and who can view setbacks as part of the process. These individuals get uncomfortable all the time, but they acknowledge their discomfort with courage. What do you admire about the person you chose? Refer to Appendix E7 for the Life Athlete Using Setbacks to Improve Future Behavior Activity.

> How you think about your distress helps to determine its impact on your behavior!

Exercise

Moving beyond weight loss, exercise and a physically-active lifestyle are often heralded as the most significant behavioral predictors for long-term weight maintenance. Successful maintainers often decrease their total caloric expenditure from physical activity following active weight loss; however, they still expend approximately fifty percent more calories per week when compared to regainers. Weight regain is also significantly influenced by exercise self-efficacy. I know, another big word—you're going to be so smart when you're done with this book. Self-efficacy describes how confident you are in your ability to maintain an effort level necessary to meet exercise goals under various circumstances. Self-efficacy represents a psychological component related to long-term weight and health goal achievement, but it is not often addressed in terms of eating and exercise. That is why we thought it so important to include such an expansive section related to the psychology of health-related goals.

Use it or Lose it: The cognitive distortions presented earlier in this chapter can weaken even the strongest athlete's resolve to exercise or eat well and compromise their sense of confidence in their ability to meet the demands of their goals. The old adage "use it or lose it" applies in the context of cognitive and behavior change. You must pursue this vigilantly if you expect it to stick. Refer to Appendix E8 for the Life Athlete Exercise Activity.

Develop Commitment through a Strong Support System

Engrained patterns of behavior require significant effort and practice to replace. Remember the words "intention" and "deliberate." Among individuals who unsuccessfully maintain weight loss, a commonly expressed barrier is the perceived effort it takes to maintain and the ease with which old habits return. In fact, seventy-five percent of regainers in one study reported maintenance being significantly difficult or impossible to achieve.

Individuals who have maintained for longer periods of time, upwards of six years, report the level of attention necessary to devote to maintenance is far lower than those who have been maintaining for two to three years. As a result, longer protocols are suggested to address the level of support apparently necessary to facilitate longer-term maintenance, and when support contacts remain constant, even at a monthly or bi-monthly interval scheme, participants show maintenance of sixty- to eighty-percent of their behaviors learned.

This is the reason The Diet Doc advocates for long-term contact with its clients. While the skills necessary for effective weight loss and long-term health are being learned through the interaction and collaboration that is built into the consulting model that we offer, every step of the process is focused on the overriding goal of sustainability and empowerment.

Of course this does not mean that you are dependent upon a weight-loss consultant for the rest of your life. What it does demonstrate is the higher level of personal awareness that you have built and the vigilance with which you are pursing your goal of lifetime health and a balanced relationship with food, with the understanding that it will take consistent and persistent effort and support.

Be a Lifer: I am told often by new clients that they have made the decision not to tell anyone that they are on a diet. This actually makes me very happy. First, I don't want them to feel they are on a diet. Secondly, telling others you are on a diet can bring unwanted attention. As the Diet Doc advocates a change in your health-related behaviors, the program is much less a diet and more a life transformation. I wouldn't propose that they keep their goals a secret, but instead, when asked about their new behaviors, be proud to say they have decided to be as healthy as possible, permanently. Refer to Appendix E9 for the Life Athlete Develop Commitment Through a Strong Support System Activity.

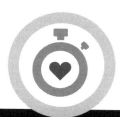

SECTION 4:
Metabolic Transformation Scholar

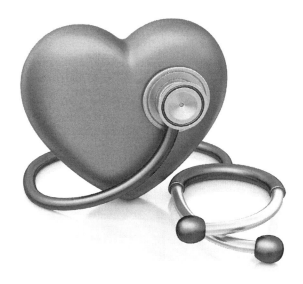

CHAPTER SIXTEEN

Special Insert:
Permanent Weight-Loss Key Concepts

Time to Put on the Big Boy Pants!

The Rapid Results Guide, meal exchange list, and recipes are resources designed to lock you onto a path of early results. They help you break into faster fat loss while you're learning the process. Within a couple of weeks, though, the training wheels have to come off and we need to establish a track of information for long-term success. It's time to learn how nutrition works and the unique capabilities of your body. It will take a little work, but with the foundation you've already built, it's really not that difficult. Many fad diets boast a tagline, "No calorie counting, no weighing, no measuring!" Guess what? Studies have shown that the single greatest common habit of those who succeed with permanent weight loss is food tracking. The exchange list provided a template, now think of it as an opportunity to expand your options and to be more flexible—not a bad thing at all. There are hundreds of food count websites online, books, and even Web apps to help, but you'll need a numeric goal to target. I'll include a modified version of the original Diet Doc Rx, but we've also created one for people who are more active.

The Diet Doc Rx

I designed the use of macronutrient tracking almost two decades ago to give clients—and myself!—the ability to be flexible with food choices. It's a budget; it's simple math. We have found over the years that some people need to start with a template and are more comfortable following an exact meal plan. That's why the Rapid Results Guide and meal exchange lists were created for *50 Days*, but you're going to advance and need a progression. So...drum roll...here is the new-and-improved Diet Doc Rx and an advanced version for super-duper-active, athletic readers. We expect everyone to be more active after reading this book, but if you're starting from a moderately sedentary lifestyle, stick to the original version. If you're training aggressively, you'll need the Metabolic Inferno chart.

Everyone is different metabolically and these charts may need to be modified for some readers. The Diet Doc Rx was created for the general population with a moderate activity level with a goal of losing one- to two-pounds per week. You might lose five- to ten-pounds the first week due to glycogen and water loss, but one- to two-pounds each week thereafter is a safe, quick pace. Other diets may promise faster results, but when we're talking about actual fat loss, losing much more would likely be unsafe, cause metabolic suppression, and set you up for rapid regain.

If, despite following your suggested macronutrient intake perfectly, eating the best food selections as described, and using the methods in this book, you are not obtaining the desired results, you might need to make an adjustment. First, if you are not losing weight fast enough (one- to two-pounds per week) make sure you're eating at the low end of your macronutrient range. If you are losing too rapidly, make sure you're eating at the high end. If you're still losing too fast, add twenty grams of carbohydrates to your daily intake for a week and reassess your results. Keep adding until you are losing at the desired rate. If you are still losing too slowly, even at the low end of your suggested chart totals, drop your daily intake of carbs by ten grams for a week and reassess. Repeat weekly until you are losing weight at the appropriate rate.

The Launching Point

As discussed earlier, your body has many sources of energy to draw from. Once calories are decreased below what is necessary (basal metabolic rate), the caloric deficit must be made up from another source, external or internal. Though we would all like body fat to be used, a percentage of energy is taken from almost every available source. The most readily available is blood sugar and then liver glycogen (stored carbs). These are dynamic, easy-to-access energy stores that are immediately used when needed.

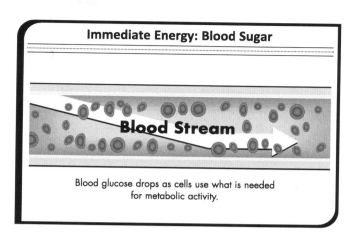

Immediate Energy: Blood Sugar

Blood Stream

Blood glucose drops as cells use what is needed for metabolic activity.

Muscle glycogen is a large source of stored energy, but its primary purpose is for muscle contraction and is not easily retrieved for maintenance calorie needs. Between meals, body fat is released from body fat cells, but only as much as is needed. Since your caloric intake is moderately lower than your body needs on a daily basis, you now require a secondary source of energy. Your body is first going to access blood sugar, liver glycogen, and a moderate amount of available muscle glycogen (especially if you work out)—all "carb" sources. The Diet Doc Rx chart is designed to take a large portion of the caloric deficit from carbohydrates so that as you continue using blood sugar and glycogen, you will eventually (within two- to four-days) be as depleted as your brain will safely allow. Blood sugar levels are critical

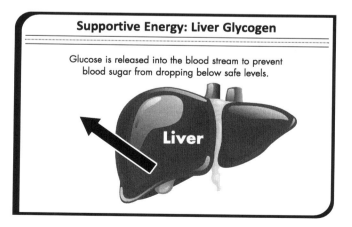

Supportive Energy: Liver Glycogen

Glucose is released into the blood stream to prevent blood sugar from dropping below safe levels.

Liver

The New Diet Doc Rx (Personal Macronutrient Range)

Height	Men: (Grams per day)	Women: (Grams per day)
Under 5'		
Protein	110 - 120	70 - 80
Carbohydrates	140 - 150	100 - 110
Fat	40 - 45	25 - 30
(Calories)	(1,360 - 1,485)	(905 – 1,030)
5' - 5'4"		
Protein	120 - 130	80 - 90
Carbohydrates	150 - 160	110 - 120
Fat	45 - 50	25 - 30
(Calories)	(1,485 - 1,610)	(985 - 1,110)
5'5" - 5'8"		
Protein	130 - 140	90 - 100
Carbohydrates	160 - 170	120 - 130
Fat	50 - 55	30 - 35
(Calories)	(1,610 - 1,735)	(1,110 - 1,235)
5'9" - 6'		
Protein	140 - 150	100 - 110
Carbohydrates	170 - 180	130 - 140
Fat	55 - 60	30 - 35
(Calories)	(1,735 - 1,860)	(1,190 - 1,315)
6'1" - 6'4"		
Protein	150 - 160	110 - 120
Carbohydrates	180 - 190	140 - 150
Fat	60 - 65	35 - 40
(Calories)	(1,860 - 1,985)	(1,315 - 1,440)
Over 6'5"		
Protein	160 - 170	120 - 130
Carbohydrates	190 - 200	150 - 160
Fat	65 - 70	35 - 40
(Calories)	(1,985 - 2,110)	(1,395 - 1,520)

The Diet Doc Metabolic Inferno Rx (Personal Macronutrient Range)

Height	Men: (Grams per day)	Women: (Grams per day)
Under 5'		
Protein	120 - 130	80 - 90
Carbohydrates	140 - 150	110 - 120
Fat	40 - 45	25 - 30
(Calories)	(1,400 - 1,525)	(985 – 1,110)
5' - 5'4"		
Protein	140 - 150	100 - 110
Carbohydrates	160 - 170	130 - 140
Fat	45 - 50	30 - 35
(Calories)	(1,605 - 1,730)	(1,190 - 1,315)
5'5" - 5'8"		
Protein	160 - 170	120 - 130
Carbohydrates	180 - 190	150 - 160
Fat	50 - 55	35 - 40
(Calories)	(1,810 - 1,935)	(1,395 - 1,520)
5'9" - 6'		
Protein	180 - 190	140 - 150
Carbohydrates	200 - 210	170 - 180
Fat	55 - 60	40 - 45
(Calories)	(2,015 - 2,140)	(1,600 - 1,725)
6'1" - 6'4"		
Protein	200 - 210	160 - 170
Carbohydrates	220 - 230	190 - 200
Fat	60 - 65	45 - 50
(Calories)	(2,220 - 2,345)	(1,805 - 1,930)
Over 6'5"		
Protein	220 - 230	180 - 190
Carbohydrates	240 - 250	210 - 220
Fat	65 - 70	50 - 55
(Calories)	(2,425 - 2,550)	(2,010 - 2,135)

Personal Macronutrient Rx

_____ grams of protein per day

_____ grams of carbohydrate per day

_____ grams of fat per day

MEAL	TIME	PORTION SIZE	FOOD CONSUMED PER MEAL	TOTAL GRAMS		
				Pro	Carb	Fat
1						
2						
3						
4						
5						
6						
			TOTALS FOR DAY			

to the brain and closely monitored. If you experience substantial cravings or feel weak and shaky, you might need to increase your carbs a bit, or at least eat your next meal or snack a little sooner. Make sure you stay well hydrated and get plenty of sleep. You can avoid transitional headaches and inordinate hunger if you keep meals on schedule and keep drinking plenty of water. Since this is not a low-carb diet, any discomfort you feel should be brief as your body catches back up with these secondary energy sources. Think of it is a rite of passage that leads to success, but you should be able to get through it easily.

You now have reached a level of carbohydrate depletion that opens a door to significant body-fat usage. If you raid the fridge at this point, you'll refill your muscle and liver glycogen, as well as your blood glucose (sugar), and you'll have to start over. Unfortunately, this is a pattern of many dieters. Three or four days might go well, and then a binge can send you back to the starting block both physically and mentally. In reality, you're depleting and repleting carb stores without much alteration in body fat. Though you might be eating well most of the time, you won't lose weight.

If you stay within your macronutrient ranges once moderately carb depleted, a great shift takes place.

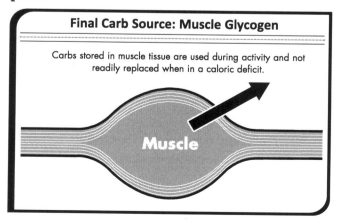

Final Carb Source: Muscle Glycogen

Carbs stored in muscle tissue are used during activity and not readily replaced when in a caloric deficit.

Muscle

Since you're still consuming carbohydrates, this depletion process is somewhat slow—and therefore safe and tolerable. But, you are still in a calorie deficit and without stored carbs to make up the difference your body finally heads for body fat. Two things will now happen that allow for immediate and consistent body fat loss. Body fat cells start releasing fatty acids and glycerol, the products of stored body fat. Once in the blood stream, some is used directly by certain types of cells for energy (lipolysis) while some is converted into glucose. This mechanism is called gluconeogenesis—literally the creation of new glucose. Now blood sugar levels come back up to a consistent level and you should see energy increase and hunger decrease. As long as you're consistent with your suggested food intake totals, you're now making up the majority of the caloric deficit by turning your body fat into usable carbohydrates. By learning how to take advantage of this inherent survival mechanism you're going to lose body fat without the suffering fad diets often cause.

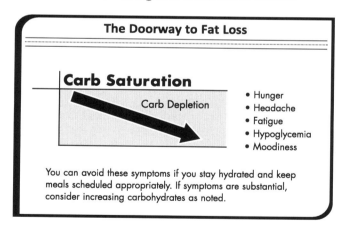

The Doorway to Fat Loss

Carb Saturation

Carb Depletion

- Hunger
- Headache
- Fatigue
- Hypoglycemia
- Moodiness

You can avoid these symptoms if you stay hydrated and keep meals scheduled appropriately. If symptoms are substantial, consider increasing carbohydrates as noted.

Another way of explaining it is that the brain needs a constant supply of glucose. In order to make sure glucose levels aren't too high or too low, the brain directs the pancreas to produce more glucagon (a hormone that increases blood sugar) or insulin (a hormone that stores blood sugar). Fat loss or fat gain isn't the primary goal of the body with food; it's an indirect effect based on what hormone—glucagon or insulin—is present most often. Too much carbohydrate in one meal results in insulin being released in large enough supply to store new body fat. Too little carbohydrate and the body goes into retrieval mode, looking for an alternative energy. When too much carbohydrate is present and insulin runs rampant, we store the glucose in our liver and muscle, (meaning we have to once again deplete that carbohydrate to begin burning body fat maximally), and some of the blood glucose gets directly pulled into fat cells and stored as fat. Does the term "yo-yo dieting" come to mind?

Keep in mind that each gram of glycogen holds approximately three times its weight in water. A by-product of cellular metabolism is also water. The first week of decreasing your body's level of stored carbohydrates, and beginning the process of losing body fat, will result in a large amount of water loss. It isn't uncommon for someone to lose five- to ten-pounds in the first week. The second week will be a truer reflection of how much body fat is being lost.

Cheat Meals, Splurge Meals, Relaxed Meals...Fun Meals!

We actually debated like a focus group to come up with the name of the *indulgent* meal. We want you to have a *relaxed* meal once a week where you don't necessarily count every gram and you eat enough to make that day closer to a calorie-neutral day rather than another day in a calorie deficit. If we call it a *cheat* meal, will you subconsciously feel evil and wrong as your fork pierces the chocolate lava cake? If we call it a *splurge* meal, will you think of it like a shopping spree and try to cram as much in as you can before the timer stops? We ended up liking *relaxed* meal a little more, so at least maybe you'll slow down and enjoy it. I tend to eat like my Doberman—she can swallow a thirty-two ounce steak and look at me with eyebrows raised, *what else ya got, big boy?*

You need ground rules; we know. This isn't a relaxed day or a lay-on-the-couch-moaning relaxed meal after visiting every buffet in town. If you're on track with your normal meals and you're losing at the pace described, you should consider having one meal per week where you enjoy foods you've been avoiding as not-the-best-weight-loss foods. Have a couple slices of pizza and a dessert. Enjoy a steak and potato and even a dinner roll. Eat a moderate amount and enjoy it without guilt. You'll be replacing your normal dinner and possibly a snack, so the calorie overage isn't that great—you might not even make it over your metabolic rate.

We're not just push-overs; a bigger meal can help your efforts. First, you need that boost in food intake so that your body doesn't continue in a chronic calorie deficit for too long. Second, you get a nice break from the deficit and the feeling of being deprived. You might not think you need these pauses, but chronic depletion can sneak up on you and this short hiatus can make you less prone to binging.

A routine off-plan meal—which is part of the plan, so it's really not off plan—is also a great training device. If you get used to eating "normal," or "bad," food, without going overboard in quantity, it helps develop a more moderate mindset. Most of us all tend to slip into all-or-none crisis mode, and staying away from *those* foods only make us want them more. Exposing yourself to decadent food can desensitize you to extreme reactions like wanting to eat all the sugary food in the house. Speaking of exposing, a couple famous classic writers claimed their best work was written naked...maybe we should make this a really relaxed meal!

So where was I? You have the flexibility of a floating relaxed meal to use for special occasions. Plan for that birthday party or football game. Work on control, but enjoy!

Carbs, Carbs, and More Carbs

Carbohydrates provide most of the energy for our bodies most of the time. Because they require the least amount of energy to break down, they are the easiest of the macronutrients to digest and be converted to glucose. Carb sources are loosely described as sugar, starch, or fiber, and these are commonly categorized as simple or complex carbohydrates. You might think of simple carbohydrates as junk food, like soda and candy, and complex carbs as whole foods, such as potatoes, pasta, and bread. This type of labeling leads to the assumption that a particular food is either good or bad when actually there is more of a continuum.

Glucose is the smallest form of sugar that the human body uses for energy. Whatever type of carbohydrate you consume, the end result of digestion is glucose whenever possible. The pathway of digestion that leads to glucose can affect our energy levels, mental acuity, physical functioning, and even athletic performance. The source of carbohydrates you choose will make a difference.

You might recognize the names of various forms of sugar: glucose, lactose, fructose, maltose, dextrose, sucrose, and so on. Each one of these carbohydrates has a different level of molecular complexity. Those that are structurally simple are quick to digest. When dieting, this isn't always the best choice. Carbs with a more complex molecular structure are harder to digest and take longer to move through the digestion process. That can be good for hunger prevention and blood sugar stability. The *Glycemic Index* is a scale that ranks carbohydrate foods by comparing digestion rate. It reveals the simplicity or complexity of the sugar, starch, and fiber that make up carbohydrates.

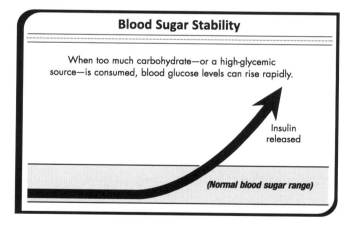

Blood Sugar Stability

When too much carbohydrate—or a high-glycemic source—is consumed, blood glucose levels can rise rapidly.

Insulin released

(Normal blood sugar range)

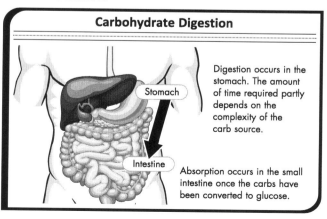

Carbohydrate Digestion

Stomach

Digestion occurs in the stomach. The amount of time required partly depends on the complexity of the carb source.

Intestine

Absorption occurs in the small intestine once the carbs have been converted to glucose.

Weird Asides— But You Would Ask Anyway

Two caveats that need explanation are fiber and sugar alcohol. The popularity of low-carb diets has led people to believe that fiber and sugar alcohol are "free" and don't need considered. Fiber, though it is digested slower, is a carbohydrate. Any that doesn't end up digested in the stomach can be broken down in the large intestine and absorbed in different forms. So, while fibrous carbs are good, healthy sources, they are still carbohydrates. Fiber is necessary, but it's not free.

An interesting carbohydrate source that the FDA hasn't classified firmly is sugar alcohol, or polyphenols. Used in some baked products and prevalent in protein bars, sugar alcohol (usually in the form of glycerine or glycerol) is actually part of a fat molecule. Being calorically similar to a carbohydrate, but structurally coming from a fat molecule, it is digested very slowly without causing a fast rise in blood sugar. Originally, this—and maybe lobbying by the low-carb diet industry— led the FDA to not even require listing it on the label. I warned you this was weird. I'm assuming the rationale was *we don't know what it is, so we'll just ignore it*. (I see parallels to the 24,000-page tax code.)

Whether due to lobbying efforts by the low-carb food producers, or legitimately due to the reduced danger to diabetics (since it doesn't cause a substantial increase in blood sugar), sugar alcohol was allowed to fly under the radar. When the outcry was loud enough, the FDA started requiring them to be rightly listed on labels as part of "total carbohydrates," but they continue to allow fiber and polyphenols to be deducted to create a new category: net carbs. These carbs are there and need to be counted. Don't deduct fiber, and you can ignore "net carb" counts; track "total carbohydrates." Now you see why the U.S. doesn't rank in the top twenty in math.

Alcoholic beverages are similar but labels don't even provide the courtesy of the "net carb" count. Take a look at any low-carb light beer and you'll find near-zero protein and fat counts, a low carbohydrate count, but calories listed at a much higher level than if you did the math. (Protein and carbs have four calories per gram and fat has nine.) The missing calories are uncounted sugar alcohol. Wine and hard liquor contain roughly four- to six-grams of "carbs" per ounce, though they'll be often listed as just one. I put carbs in quotes because they're not classified as such, but they have almost the exact same caloric level (actually a bit more) and they're used even faster. That light beer that you've been downing at a cost of only seven- to nine-grams of carbs is really about twenty- to twenty-five per bottle. I know, I know… pull yourself together. There's always the relaxed meal. Save room for a tall, cold one.

I Knew I Should Have Taken Organic Chemistry!

When you consume a high-glycemic carbohydrate such as white bread, a banana, a baked potato, or candy, little digestion needs to take place. The carbohydrate passes through the stomach quickly and enters the small intestine. Absorption occurs in the small intestine where uptake is rapid. Since your brain closely monitors blood sugar levels, a fast increase triggers your pancreas to release the hormone insulin. Remember, insulin is the storage hormone that shuttles blood glucose where necessary or to be stored if there is no immediate need.

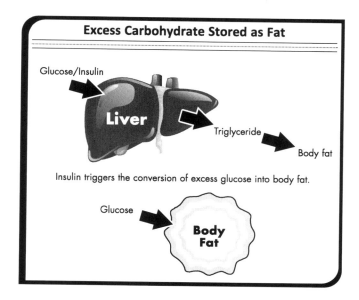

Excess Carbohydrate Stored as Fat

Glucose/Insulin

Liver

Triglyceride

Body fat

Insulin triggers the conversion of excess glucose into body fat.

Glucose

Body Fat

If too much carb has been consumed at one meal, or the source is simple enough to trigger a large amount of insulin, the liver will convert the blood sugar into triglycerides (fat) to be ultimately stored. Insulin also triggers body fat cells to simply pull excess glucose in to be converted directly to body fat.

None of the aforementioned high-glycemic carb sources have fat in them, but a large portion of the carbs can be converted to body fat due to the effect of insulin. Unfortunately, the problems don't stop there. Whether by storage or utilization, blood glucose levels return to normal and your brain tells your pancreas to stop releasing insulin. Even with the process stopped, a certain amount of insulin remains active in the bloodstream until it is resynthesized. This means more glucose will be removed, dropping blood sugar below a normal level. We all know how that feels. You can end up tired, as in the case of the after-lunch dosing, or not wanting to unpeel yourself from the couch after dinner.

As blood sugar levels plummet, your brain sends out powerful hormonal messengers to signal hunger. Ever eat something and end up even hungrier a short while later? Too much of a drop can cause severe symptoms such as hypoglycemia.

This whole process wreaks havoc on body composition, energy levels, and it might start with a "fat-free" food or at least one that didn't seem unhealthy. It could be just too much carbohydrate at one time, even if it was a good choice. When the carbohydrate cravings kick in due to lower blood sugar levels, it's easy to start the process all over again. This is a powerful biochemical reaction. Massive, seemingly uncontrollable binges are birthed by insulin-induced blood sugar drops. Many of us live on this roller coaster and don't realize that we're the ones causing it! *I just have a slow metabolism,* or *you just naturally gain more body fat as you get older* become self-deluded mantras that prevent us from living a leaner, healthier life.

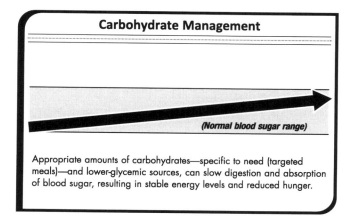

Carbohydrate Management

(Normal blood sugar range)

Appropriate amounts of carbohydrates—specific to need (targeted meals)—and lower-glycemic sources, can slow digestion and absorption of blood sugar, resulting in stable energy levels and reduced hunger.

What if you chose a carbohydrate on the other end of the glycemic index, such as a grapefruit, a bowl of oatmeal, or even a salad? These carb sources have different molecular configurations—much more complex. When they hit your stomach, digestion takes longer to break them into usable glucose molecules. Since this process takes more time, the resulting glucose enters the small intestine and is absorbed more gradually, blood sugar levels rise more slowly, and a major insulin increase is prevented. Just by changing the carb source, you have decreased the potential for the creation of new body fat, and your energy rises over the next couple of hours instead of dipping quickly. A great side effect is that hunger is dramatically reduced because blood glucose levels are stable.

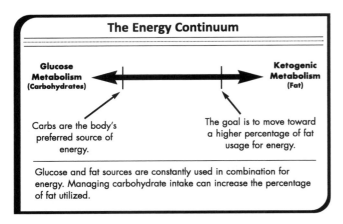

The Energy Continuum

Glucose Metabolism (Carbohydrates) ←——————————→ **Ketogenic Metabolism (Fat)**

Carbs are the body's preferred source of energy.

The goal is to move toward a higher percentage of fat usage for energy.

Glucose and fat sources are constantly used in combination for energy. Managing carbohydrate intake can increase the percentage of fat utilized.

During a client consultation I was asked, "So, keeping insulin low is the whole key?" There are so many swirling factors occurring at once, and so many chemical actions depend on or affect one other, but I had to simply admit, "Yes." Insulin and glucagon are the two opposing hormones that keep blood sugar either increasing or decreasing to normal levels. If we need more glucose, glucagon is released and through all the machinations discussed, we end up losing fat. When there is excess glucose, insulin is produced to bring blood sugar down, and part, or most of it, is stored as fat. We're either storing or retrieving.

When carbs are eaten in appropriate amounts, insulin is held at bay and glucagon is present more often. Voila: body fat loss. An oversimplified explanation, but it is the *whole key*.

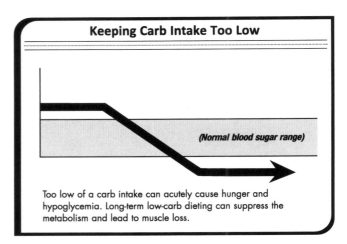

Keeping Carb Intake Too Low

(Normal blood sugar range)

Too low of a carb intake can acutely cause hunger and hypoglycemia. Long-term low-carb dieting can suppress the metabolism and lead to muscle loss.

Does the Glycemic Index Really Matter?

Many individuals cruise through early dieting success only to be slammed with massive cravings. I have a friend who claims to be addicted to cookies. "I just can't have one or I'll lose control," he tells me. I think we've all been there: four or five days into a diet we find ourselves at the bottom of a gallon of ice cream or lying on the couch with our pants unsnapped after cleaning out the pantry. *I've already blown it; I might as well finish the Lucky Charms, eat the last few tortilla chips…what the heck; Susie wasn't going to finish her Halloween candy anyway; I'll polish that off just to get it out of the house and start my diet again Monday.*

Sometimes that one taste of sugar can send us into a tailspin behaviorally, but if we consume a lot of it at once, the physical carnage of insulin begins. Blood sugar levels are quickly pulled down leaving us to face serious, real cravings. The same result can occur, though, if we don't consume enough carbohydrate. Anyone who has followed their peers over the low-carb-diet cliff knows how horrible it feels to walk around in a low-blood-sugar daze. Both missteps carry the same risk. A badly-timed high-glycemic carb, or going too long without carbohydrates, can lead to unnecessary hunger, an energy crash, or a head-first dive into a binge.

Sample Glycemic Index Selections

The glycemic index rates the speed of carbohydrate digestion and the subsequent impact on blood sugar elevation. A zero rating would indicate no carbohydrate present, while 100 was designed to be the highest rating—that of table sugar. Some foods were later determined to increase blood glucose even faster and rank higher than 100.

	Glycemic Index Value	Serving Size	Grams of Carbs per Serving
CEREALS AND BREADS			
All Bran®	30	1/2 cup	15
Oatmeal (rolled oats)	42	1/2 cup (dry)	27
Oatbran bread	47	1 slice	18
Rye bread	58	1 slice	14
Raisin Bran™	61	1/2 cup	19
Pancakes	67	2-4"	58
Special K™	69	1 cup	21
Bagel, white	72	1	70
Grape Nuts™	75	1/4 cup	22
Shredded Wheat™	75	1 cup	30
English muffin	77	1	14
Whole wheat bread	77	1 slice	12
White bread	80	1 slice	14
Crispix™	87	1 cup	25
Rice Krispies™	87	1 cup	21
Corn Flakes™	92	1 cup	26
SNACKS			
Potato chips	57	2 oz	18
Blueberry muffin	59	3.5 oz	47
Tortilla chips	63	2 oz	30
Protein bar	74	3.6 oz	50
Soda crackers	74	5	15
Rice cake	82	1	7
Pretzels	83	1 oz	20

	Glycemic Index Value	Serving Size	Grams of Carbs per Serving
COMMON "STARCH" SOURCES FOR MEALS			
Pasta, wheat	32	1 cup	40
Pasta, white	38	1 cup	40
Sweet potato	44	5 oz	25
Rice, brown	50	1/2 cup	17
Rice, long-grain	61	1/2 cup	18
Rice, white	87	1/2 cup	28
Potato, baked	85	5 oz	30
FRUIT			
Cherries	22	1/2 cup	10
Grapefruit	25	1/2	11
Apple	38	4 oz	15
Pear	38	4 oz	11
Orange	42	4 oz	11
Peach	42	4 oz	11
Grapes	46	1 cup	24
Banana	52	4 oz	24
Raisins	64	1/2 cup	44
Cantaloupe	65	4 oz	6
Pineapple	66	4 oz	10
Watermelon	72	4 oz	6
VEGETABLES			
Broccoli	15	1 cup	5
Cauliflower	15	1 cup	5
Lettuce	15	1 cup	2
Carrots	47	1 cup	10
Peas	48	1/2 cup	10
Corn	60	1/2 cup	18

(*The New Glucose Revolution*, by Jennie Brand-Miller is recommended for further values and understanding of the glycemic index.)

Your Body is a Wonderland

In case you didn't know, that is a song title. If you have to explain a joke, it's not funny—I get it—but I couldn't risk anyone thinking I'm a complete weirdo. And the lyric fits: your own gastrointestinal system actually gives you a carbohydrate safety net, if you know how to use it. So far, I've given examples of low- and high-glycemic carb digestive pathways, but the glycemic index is a continuum—every food fits in somewhere. Choosing carb sources low on the glycemic index will help reduce hunger, but what if you *really* want a higher-glycemic carb?

Protein and fat molecules are larger than carbohydrates. Digesting them can take hours. The valve (pyloric sphincter) between the stomach and small intestine will stay closed as digestion takes place, opening only one- to three-times per minute while the food is broken down. If you eat a carb source in combination with fat and protein, the carbohydrate gets caught up in the slowed digestive process. In short, a carb eaten alone will be digested and absorbed much faster than one eaten with fat and protein. The vast majority of the time, slowed absorption of our carbs is a good thing!

There are a couple of things to keep in mind, though. One is the practical side of nutrition. Don't misunderstand and think that every meal or snack has to have a *perfect* balance of nutrients or that you can never eat a carbohydrate source alone. Secondly, as you learned regarding targeted meals, there are times where a stand-alone carb can be the perfect snack. Context is important when choosing.

Goin' Old School with Fat

Explaining the difference between good fat and bad fat used to be revolutionary. Today you can probably learn everything you need to know from a fish oil advertisement, but let's cover some basics. In terms of dietary fat, think saturated and unsaturated. Saturated fats most commonly come from animal sources such as beef, pork, dairy products, eggs, and poultry. Products made with these animal fats—such as butter, cream, and many others—are also saturated. Some have a great deal more or less fat than others. For example, fish, chicken, and turkey breast have dramatically less than beef.

The problems with saturated fats lie primarily in their structure. They are much larger and more stable than unsaturated fats and therefore harder to break down. Saturated fats circulate in the blood stream longer, create higher blood cholesterol levels, lead to atherosclerosis, and much of it ends up being stored as body fat.

You might have heard the term "trans-fat." A fat can be classified either as a cis- or a trans-fat depending on its chemical structure. Trans-fats in general are those that are solid at room temperature and are used in cheap food processing. Your cell membranes are made up of fat molecules that create receptor sites—like ports—for nutrients and chemicals to be shuttled inside the cell. Trans-fats are rotated and stuck in a backward position that doesn't allow transport to occur. The cell can't function properly. Trans-fats have been linked to cancer as well as heart disease for this reason.

Unsaturated fats are found mainly in plant sources such as olive oil, canola oil, flaxseed oil, grapeseed oil, borage oil, some nuts, and in some fish like salmon. Molecularly, unsaturated fats are smaller, less stable, and easier to break down. Unsaturated fats actually have some important health benefits and can help you lose body fat. They contain specific essential fatty acids, which have been the subjects of significant research during the last couple of decades. Each essential fatty acid has unique properties beneficial to the human body. Notice they're called "essential," a biological term meaning your body can't produce them, so your diet needs to supply them.

Seriously...Good?

You might have heard the terms "good fat" and "bad fat." Some essential fatty acids are the building blocks for specific hormones that control fat loss and storage and the potential for muscle gain and loss. Yes, your body produces hormones that control how much body fat you can lose or gain and how much muscle you can gain or lose. Your body needs unsaturated fats (essential fatty acids) to create many of these hormones, such as testosterone. People who consume a no- or low-fat diet start producing less of the hormones that promote body fat loss and muscle gain, especially if body fat levels are low. Conversely, people who consume twenty- to thirty-percent of their calories from unsaturated fat start producing more of these hormones. With an increase in your hormonal base, you can burn more body fat and build more muscle than normal. Research has demonstrated these positive blood chemistry changes can lead to decreased cholesterol and increased athletic performance. A little of the right dietary fat goes a long way.

I have witnessed dramatic decreases in cholesterol and LDL's (low-density lipoproteins, or "bad fat" in the bloodstream) by increasing unsaturated

fat, managing carbohydrates better, and adding exercise. I have to qualify this, though, with what I see as a very practical aspect of body fat loss and dieting. Most people who are overweight and eating a poor diet consume too much refined carbohydrate and too much saturated fat. A few hold-overs from the low-fat craze are eating healthy and fall into the need-more-good-fat category, but most of us are killing ourselves on both ends. Many achieve the best health and results by eliminating saturated fats and increasing unsaturated fats while keeping carbs in check. You can't leave out carbohydrate control when discussing cholesterol.

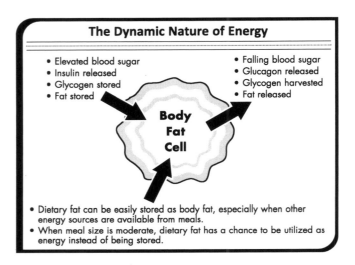

The Dynamic Nature of Energy

- Elevated blood sugar
- Insulin released
- Glycogen stored
- Fat stored

Body Fat Cell

- Falling blood sugar
- Glucagon released
- Glycogen harvested
- Fat released

- Dietary fat can be easily stored as body fat, especially when other energy sources are available from meals.
- When meal size is moderate, dietary fat has a chance to be utilized as energy instead of being stored.

Up to eighty percent of your body's cholesterol is produced in your liver as a result of sugar and runaway insulin. Recall that excess carbohydrates result in a conversion to cholesterol and fat. By substantially reducing saturated fat and recommending a moderate intake of unsaturated fats while controlling carbohydrate levels, I have watched hypercholesterolemic clients (those whose livers produce a significantly larger amount of cholesterol) lower their cholesterol levels and manage them so well that, under the supervision of their physicians, they have been able to eliminate the use of cholesterol-reducing medications. A client referred to me decreased his blood triglycerides from over 900 to 90 in 3 months using our original *Metabolic Transformation* program along with weight training and cardiovascular exercise. A triglyceride level of 900—his poor heart was pumping sludge, not blood! Diet should be the cornerstone of any cholesterol management program, not an afterthought. If you need medication, then take it; heart disease is serious business, but cholesterol-lowering medication shouldn't be viewed as an excuse to not lose weight and exercise.

Draining Those Pesky Fat Cells

A point that must be understood is how dynamic fat is in the body. We constantly store triglycerides in adipose (fat) cells at meals and release it as energy is needed. Fat is used for up to sixty percent of the body's energy needs at rest. It can be surprising how easily the body stores dietary fat as body fat. Dietary fat is the easiest nutrient for your body to store as body fat. As digested dietary fat is carried past adipose cells in the bloodstream through capillaries, adipose cells simply intake the fat to be stored. Recall the small three-percent thermic effect of fat. I know that may sound contradictory after making such a big deal about carbohydrates, but don't throw the baby out with the bath water. It is a fact that dietary fat is easier to store as body fat than carbohydrates when calorie intake is *more than your body can digest and use at that particular meal.* You need to keep carbs lower and in control to get accelerated fat-loss potential as described, but keep everything in perspective. Food volume is step one, targeted meal formatting is step two, carb quality and quantity is step three, and then fat intake

closely follows in importance.

Calorie intake is still always the first step. Total calorie consumption is taken care of by eating within the boundaries of your personal macronutrient range, even as you might be adjusting to tailor your plan. If you're taking in a moderate amount of fat, even unsaturated fats, a great deal of it can end up stored as fat if carbs or overall calories are too high. But, if your overall calorie intake is lower than your metabolic rate requires, you'll end up using that dietary fat as well as stored fat between meals.

So, if too much dietary fat ends up being stored as body fat, why not just eliminate it completely? It seems we've had this conversation about carbs! Recall that essential fatty acids play a role in hormone production as well as cellular repair, immune function, and many other life processes. Another key reason is the focus on keeping blood sugar moderated. Fat takes longer to digest and slows the digestion and assimilation of carbohydrates, so insulin spiking is less of a problem. This type of fat intake has merit, but only if the percentages are representative of an overall calorie intake that's low enough to cause a caloric deficit—if your goal is to lose. As already discussed, the relationship between fats and carbohydrates is very important. If fat intake, for example, is twenty-five percent of the total calories instead of fifteen percent, a little lower carbohydrate intake will be necessary to accommodate the additional dietary fat. But be careful; lowering the carbohydrates might then make the practicality of food intake difficult, and energy levels can drop. Thus, a slightly lower fat intake, allowing for more carbohydrates, might be helpful. Some flexibility between carbohydrates and fat is fine, and you should feel comfortable trying different combinations as long as you stay within both ranges.

Saturated Fat Reducing Tips

1) *Use non-stick cooking spray to reduce fat or use unsaturated oils when cooking.*

2) *Boil, roast, bake, or steam food instead of frying.*

3) *Use egg whites in place of whole eggs when baking. Two egg whites equal one whole egg.*

4) *Use skim milk instead of whole or two-percent milk.*

5) *Choose low- or non-fat yogurt, mayo, and salad dressings.*

6) *Use spices and fat-free condiments, such as salsa, to spice up food.*

7) *Use applesauce or pumpkin instead of butter and/or oil in baked goods.*

8) *Make sure canned tuna, chicken, and other meats are packed in water, not oil.*

9) *Choose the leanest cuts of meat.*

10) *Trim fat from meat.*

While we're on the topic, we might as well bring up the ketogenic (low-carb) camp again. Since excess carbs are easily converted to body fat, lead to insulin-induced lethargy, and create higher risk of diabetes and heart disease, it's important to control quality and quantity. It's also imperative to make sure that carbs are low enough so they're not supplying all the energy requirements of the body—we want body fat to be used.

Ketogenic dieting is effective, there's no doubt about that. The problem is that metabolism is suppressed very quickly and weight regain is virtually impossible to avoid. One mistake people often make when trying to eliminate carbs is replacing those calories with excessive fat intake. Remember, adipose cells are just waiting to draw in new fat to store after meals. Also remember that carbs are the most protein-sparing nutrient we eat. If carbs are too low for too long, you'll lose muscle no matter how much protein you eat. Probably worse is that the brain and nervous system prefer glucose, not ketone bodies, for energy. Low energy and inefficient nervous system activity leave workouts low-key, weak, and less effective—not to mention fatigue in daily life. If you enjoy feeling lousy, having no energy, craving carbohydrates intensely, and being prone to binging, then low-carb dieting is for you. It's always tempting with the promise of the fastest fat loss, but then end results are never good for most people.

So, what's the take-home message about fat? A normal, healthy fat intake can include thirty percent or more of your calories from fat sources without a problem, but if you naturally eat less, it makes room for more carbs. If you're dieting, you might find that cutting fat intake to fifteen or twenty percent of total calories allows for a faster pace. This simply means less fat will be available for storage after meals and the amount of stored fat used between meals for energy will be coming from a faster-shrinking supply. Not to sound like I'm playing Switzerland between the two, but controlling and planning carbs and fat go hand-in-hand. Many people who obsess about carbs end up snacking on too many nuts, extra peanut butter, and other high-fat, low-carb foods, potentially increasing direct fat storage. Sometimes a little extra fat in meals can control hunger and be a good trade for some carbs. It comes down to personal preference, scheduling variables, and even body type. Don't lose sight of the big picture: dietary fat intake is a critical part of your success, but it has to be just one piece of a comprehensive plan to work.

The King of the Jungle: Protein

The amount of protein we advocate is designed to abundantly meet the body's requirements without the risk of undesirable effects. Protein is very important in creating new cells, repairing cells, and in the metabolic activities of every system in your body. If protein intake is too low, your entire body eventually suffers, even your immune system. Protein is broken down into amino acids, which are used in just about every chemical reaction that takes place within your body. Amino acids are made up of nitrogen compounds that circulate in your bloodstream and are stored as skeletal muscle and in the liver. You can live a long time without protein, and even longer with insufficient amounts of protein; your body will simply break down muscle tissue to provide what it needs. It's a great survival mechanism, but you don't want to lose any muscle.

We estimate protein requirements for active people when designing targeted meals or a comprehensive plan outline such as The Diet Doc Rx. If you aren't performing rigorous exercise at least three- to four-times per week, choose the lower end of suggested protein ranges. If you train extremely hard, or perform several sessions of cardiovascular work per week, you may benefit eating slightly above the suggested amount.

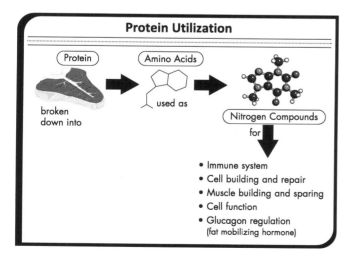

Protein Utilization

Protein → broken down into → Amino Acids → used as → Nitrogen Compounds

for
- Immune system
- Cell building and repair
- Muscle building and sparing
- Cell function
- Glucagon regulation (fat mobilizing hormone)

Please, God; not Another Chicken Breast

Every protein source has a specific amino acid profile. This means each may be higher or lower in certain amino acids than others. There are many rating scales that attempt to build a hierarchy by assigning values and deeming them high- or low-quality protein sources. These have merit, but even the highest-rated protein source is low in certain amino acids, and vice versa.

Vegetarians may have also heard that certain foods need to be combined to make a "complete protein." You're covered on two different fronts. First, digestion, absorption, and circulation keep the amino acids that you consume available for hours, and they can be augmented with other amino acids from previous or later meals. The liver also stores a small reserve of amino acids that it uses when necessary. While we're on the subject of protein and vegetarianism, I want to make sure you understand you can succeed without animal protein. We still recommend getting at least the minimal suggested protein intake in the Diet Doc Rx or your targeted meal plan for all the reasons discussed for all the reasons discussed. If you avoid protein as a vegetarian, most of your food will come from carbohydrates, causing challenges to weight loss and health in general. We have helped many vegetarians lose weight, drop their cholesterol, and regain surprising energy by trimming starch while adding a couple protein shakes per day or including another protein source acceptable to them.

The bottom line is simply to enjoy diversity of protein sources throughout your week so you take in a variety of amino acids.

Back to Hormones; I'll be Quick

Just as carbohydrates can affect your body in a positive or negative way through the modulation of the hormone insulin, protein creates a similar effect through the hormone glucagon. Insulin is released when you eat carbs; glucagon is released when you eat protein (if you don't overdo it on carbs). Insulin is a storage hormone; glucagon is a retrieval, or mobilizing, hormone. It actually promotes glucose to be used as energy. When glucose isn't present in large enough quantities (because you've been so good at limiting your carbs and sticking to your daily intake goals or meal plan!) glucagon helps mobilize body fat to be used as energy.

Insulin and glucagon represent two opposite metabolic stimuli. Insulin is present, active, and dominant if carbohydrate intake is too high—putting your body in storage mode. Glucagon is present, active, and dominant when carbohydrate intake is lower and protein intake is higher—promoting fat mobilization. Glucagon is one of several hormones that can "unlock" body fat cells and is the most powerful that is nutrition dependent. Others are more exercise dependent. When you combine the most effective nutrition and exercise to maximize these hormones, you truly are working with your body for the fastest progress.

This is a lot of information, but we wanted to include the Metabolic Transformation Scholar material to augment a deeper understanding for permanent control. Every time you come back to reference a topic, you'll pick up something new. Don't expect to soak it all up overnight, but keep coming back as you progress through your journey, and you *will* become an expert—a lean, healthy expert!

Opposing Hormones

Glucagon ←——————————————→ Insulin

- Released when blood sugar is low
- Signals body fat cells to release triglycerides
- Signals liver to convert fat to glucose
- Promotes energy stability
- Hunger decreases
- Energy increases

- Released when blood sugar is too high
- Signals body fat cells to convert glucose to fat
- Signals liver/muscle to store glucose
- Causes rebound blood sugar drop
- Hunger increases
- Energy decreases

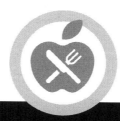

SECTION 5:
Recipes

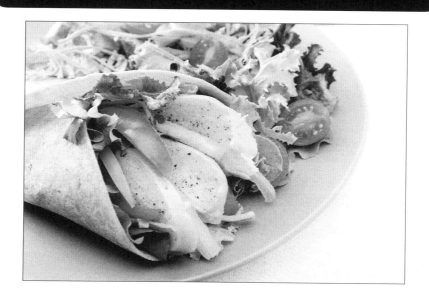

Core Recipes

Almond Crusted Chicken Salad

2 tablespoons chopped pecan halves

1 teaspoon brown sugar (not packed)

½ teaspoon light whipped butter or light buttery spread

Drop vanilla extract

2 dashes salt

1 (4 ounce) raw boneless skinless chicken breast cutlet pounded to ⅓-inch thickness

Dash each garlic powder and onion powder

2 cups chopped romaine lettuce

1 cup mixed greens

¼ cup chopped celery

2 tablespoons mandarin orange segments packed in juice, drained

1 tablespoon sweetened dried cranberries

1 tablespoon crumbled fat-free feta cheese

2 tablespoons fat-free or low-fat balsamic vinaigrette

To make the candied pecans, lay a medium piece of aluminum foil near the stove. Place pecans, sugar, and butter in a skillet; bring to medium-high heat. Stirring constantly, cook until butter and sugar have melted and mixed and pecans are coated in the mixture, about 1 minute. Remove from heat and stir in vanilla extract and a dash of salt. Spread mixture onto the foil and let cool completely.

Meanwhile, sprinkle chicken with garlic powder, onion powder, and remaining dash of salt. If needed, clean skillet. Re-spray skillet and return to medium-high heat. To pound the chicken cutlet, either lay it between two pieces of plastic wrap or place it in a sealable bag, squeeze out the air, and seal. Using a meat mallet (or heavy utensil with a flat surface), pound it until uniform in thickness. Cook chicken for about 3 minutes per side, until cooked through.

Toss lettuce with mixed greens in a bowl. Top with celery, oranges, cranberries, and cheese. Slice chicken and add to salad. Sprinkle with candied pecans. Drizzle or serve with vinaigrette.

Yield: 1 serving
Nutritional Analysis: 1 serving equals 368 calories, 16 g fat, 24.5 carbohydrate, 31 g protein
Diabetic Exchanges: 3 vegetable, 3 fat, 2 meat/cheese, 1 starch

Apple Matzo Kugel

4 sheets matzo

¼ cup light whipped butter

1 cup fat-free liquid egg substitute

1 scoop Vanilla Bean Diet Doc protein powder

¼ cup granulated white sugar

1 teaspoon vanilla extract

1 teaspoon cinnamon

½ teaspoon salt

3 cups finely-chopped Fuji apples (about 3 apples)

½ cup sweetened dried cranberries, chopped

Preheat oven to 350 degrees. Spray an 8-inch x 8-inch baking pan with nonstick spray. Break matzo into small pieces and place in a large bowl. Add just enough warm water to cover, gently pressing down to wet any pieces that float. Let soak until slightly softened, about 2 minutes. Drain well. In a small microwave-safe bowl, microwave butter for 30 seconds, or until melted.

Transfer butter to another large bowl. Add egg substitute, sugar, whey protein, vanilla extract, cinnamon, and salt. Thoroughly whisk. Add matzo and gently stir. Fold in apples and chopped cranberries. Transfer mixture to the baking pan. Bake until lightly browned and cooked through, about 45 minutes.

Yield: 8 Servings
Nutritional Analysis: 1 slice equals 170 calories, 6.5g fat, 37.5g carbs, 25.5g protein
Diabetic Exchanges: 1.5 meat/cheese, 1 fat, ½ fruit, ½ starch

Bacon Cheeseburger Casserole

1 medium-small russet potato (about 8 ounces)

4 cups chopped cauliflower

4 slices center-cut bacon or turkey bacon

2 tablespoons light whipped butter or light buttery spread

½ teaspoon salt

2 cups chopped mushrooms

1 cup chopped onion

1 10-ounce package frozen chopped spinach, thawed and squeezed dry

1/8 teaspoon black pepper

1 pound raw extra-lean ground beef (4% fat or less)

1 tablespoon yellow mustard

3 wedges Laughing Cow cheese

¼ cup ketchup

¼ cup chopped dill pickles

Preheat oven to 400 degrees. Spray a deep 8-inch x 8-inch baking pan with nonstick spray.

Bring a large pot of water to a boil. Meanwhile, peel and cube the potato.

Add potato and cauliflower to boiling water. Return to a boil, and reduce heat to medium. Cook until potato and cauliflower are very tender, 15-20 minutes.

Meanwhile, cook bacon until crispy, either in a skillet over medium heat or on a microwave-safe plate in the microwave. (Refer to package for cook time.)

Drain water and transfer potato and cauliflower to a large bowl. Add butter and ¼ teaspoon salt, and thoroughly mash.

Bring a large skillet sprayed with nonstick spray to medium-high heat. Cook and stir mushrooms and onion until softened, 5-8 minutes. Add spinach and pepper. Cook and stir until spinach is warm, about 2 minutes. Transfer veggie mixture to another large bowl. Blot away any excess moisture.

Remove skillet from heat. If needed, clean skillet. Re-spray with nonstick spray and return to medium-high heat. Add beef and sprinkle with remaining ¼ teaspoon salt.

Cook and crumble for 5-8 minutes, until cooked through.

Remove skillet from heat. Add mustard and cheese wedges, breaking the wedges into pieces, and stir until cheese has melted and is well mixed.

Chop or crumble bacon. Evenly layer ingredients in the baking pan: beef mixture, veggie mixture, bacon, and potato-cauliflower mixture.

Bake until top layer is firm, 20-25 minutes.

Spoon ketchup into one of the bottom corners of a plastic bag; snip off the tip of that corner to create a small hole, and pipe ketchup through the hole into a swirl over your casserole. (Or just drizzle the ketchup on with a spoon.)

Sprinkle with pickles, serve, and enjoy!

Yield: 6 servings
Nutritional Analysis: 1 serving equals 248 calories, 7.5 g fat, 20 g carbohydrate, 23 g protein
Diabetic Exchanges: 1.5 vegetable, 1 meat/cheese, 1 fat

Beany Proteiny Brownies

2 cans black beans, drained and rinsed

2 cups egg whites

1 cup Greek yogurt

2 packages gelatin

1.5 teaspoons baking powder

2 packages sugar-free and fat-free chocolate fudge pudding

2 teaspoons vanilla extract

1 scoop Diet Doc Vanilla Bean or Belgian Chocolate protein powder

112 grams dark chocolate chips

Preheat oven to 350 degrees. Lightly spray 9-inch x 13-inch pan with cooking spray. Combine wet ingredients in blender. Combine dry ingredients in large bowl. Pour wet ingredients into bowl and use mixer until well combined. Fold in chocolate chips. Pour into prepared pan. Bake for 30 minutes or until toothpick inserted in center comes out clean.

Yield: 12 servings
Nutritional Analysis: 1 serving equals 220 calories, 2.5 g fat, 18 g carbohydrate, 24 g protein
Diabetic Exchanges: 1.5 meat/cheese, 1 starch, ½ fat

Berry Almond Panko Tilapia

Fish:

½ cup panko breadcrumbs

2 tablespoons whole-wheat flour

2 tablespoons slivered almonds, roughly-chopped

1/8 teaspoon each garlic powder, onion powder, salt, and black pepper

¼ cup fat-free liquid egg substitute

4 4-ounce raw tilapia fillets

Sauce:

¾ cup cranberries, thawed from frozen

¼ cup orange juice

¼ cup honey Dijon mustard

1 teaspoon granulated white sugar

Preheat oven to 350 degrees. Spray a baking sheet with nonstick spray and set aside.

In a sealable plastic bag or container, combine breadcrumbs, flour, almonds, and seasonings. Seal and shake to mix. Transfer mixture to a plate, evenly spreading it out,and set aside. Place egg substitute in a shallow bowl, and set aside as well.

Make sure tilapia fillets are as dry as possible. (Blot with paper towels.) Place a fillet inegg substitute and flip to coat. Gently shake to remove excess egg substitute, and then transfer to the crumb mixture. Flip to evenly coat with crumbs, and place on the baking sheet. Repeat with remaining fillets, placing them evenly spaced on the sheet.

Bake in the oven until fish is cooked through and edges have lightly browned, 12-15 minutes.

Meanwhile, to make the sauce, bring a small nonstick pot to medium-high heat on the stove. Add cranberries and orange juice, and bring to a boil. Once boiling, reduce heat to low. Stirring occasionally, let simmer until cranberries are somewhat shriveled, about 6 minutes.

Remove from heat and allow to slightly cool. Transfer to a small blender or food processor, and add all other sauce ingredients. Pulse until smooth.

Just before serving, evenly spoon sauce over the fish, about 2 tablespoons per fillet, or serve on the side.

Yield: 4 servings
Nutritional Analysis: 1 serving equals 251 calories, 5 g fat, 20 g carbohydrate, 26.5 g protein
Diabetic Exchanges: 1.5 meat, 1 fat

Breakfast Skillet

1 frozen meatless or turkey sausage patty with about 80 calories

½ cup sliced onion

1 large portabella mushroom, roughly-chopped

⅔ cup frozen shredded hash browns

⅔ cup fat-free liquid egg substitute

½ teaspoon chopped garlic

1 wedge Laughing Cow cheese

2 tablespoons shredded fat-free cheddar cheese

Optional: salt, black pepper, chopped scallions

Prepare sausage patty on the stove in a skillet sprayed with nonstick spray or on a microwave-safe plate in the microwave. (Refer to package instructions for exact temperature and cook time.) Once cool enough to handle, crumble or chop and set aside.

Bring a skillet sprayed with nonstick spray to medium heat on the stove. Add onion and, stirring often, cook until slightly softened, about 3 minutes.

Reduce heat to medium low. Add chopped mushroom and hash browns to the skillet with the onion. Stirring occasionally, cook until mushroom pieces have softened and hash browns are hot, 5-6 minutes.

Raise heat to medium. Add cooked sausage pieces to the skillet with the veggie-hash mixture. Add egg substitute, garlic, and cheese wedge, breaking cheese wedge into pieces as you add it. Scramble until egg substitute is just cooked, about 3 minutes.

Transfer mixture to a microwave-safe plate. Sprinkle with cheddar cheese.

Microwave for 30 seconds or until cheese has just melted. If you like, season to taste with salt and pepper and top with scallions.

Yield: 1 serving
Nutritional Analysis: 1 serving equals 323 calories, 6 g fat, 28 g carbohydrate, 33 g protein
Diabetic Exchanges: 2 meat/cheese, 1 vegetable, 1 starch, 1 fat

Carrot Cake Pancakes

1 scoop Diet Doc Vanilla Bean protein powder

½ cup plain Greek yogurt

½ teaspoon cinnamon

Pinch of nutmeg

Pinch of ground ginger

Pinch of salt

½ teaspoon baking powder

2 egg whites

1 cup old fashioned oats

½ cup water

2-4 packets or ½ -1 teaspoon stevia or sweetener of choice

½ cup carrots (blended into batter) and ¼ cup carrots, grated

Optional: 2 tablespoons walnuts, chopped, 2 tablespoons golden raisins

Optional Cream Cheese Frosting:

½ cup (4 ounces) low-fat cream cheese, softened in the microwave for 30 seconds

¼ cup low-sugar or sugar-free maple syrup

Dash cinnamon

1 packet or ¼ teaspoon stevia or sweetener of your choice

Put all of the ingredients in a blender, (except for ¼ cup grated carrots and the optional add-ins), and blend until smooth. Stir in the additional grated carrots and optional add-ins (if desired).

Meanwhile, heat a nonstick griddle (or large nonstick skillet) coated with cooking spray over medium heat. Spoon about ¼ cup of batter per pancake onto griddle. Turn pancakes over when tops are covered with bubbles and edges look cooked.

To make the cream cheese frosting, whisk together the softened cream cheese, syrup, cinnamon, and stevia in a small bowl until smooth. Drizzle over pancakes while warm if desired.

Yield: 3 servings (about 3 pancakes per serving)
Nutritional Analysis: 1 serving equals 175 calories, 2 g fat, 22 g carbohydrate, 18 g protein
Diabetic Exchanges: 1 meat/cheese, 1 starch, ½ fat

Cheesy Mexican Omelet

4 egg whites

¼ teaspoon onion powder

¼ teaspoon dried basil

¼ teaspoon dried parsley flakes

¼ teaspoon celery seed

¼ cup fat-free shredded cheddar cheese

½ cup fat-free refried beans

1 ounce sliced avocado

2 tablespoons salsa

In a bowl, beat egg whites and seasonings. Lightly coat skillet with cooking spray. Add egg mixture; cook over medium heat. As eggs set, lift edges, letting uncooked portion flow underneath. When eggs are completely set, remove from the heat. Place cheese over eggs until melted.

On a separate plate spread a ½ cup fat-free refried beans in a thin layer and warm in the microwave. Place the omelet on top of the beans and top with sliced avocado and salsa.

Yield: 1 serving
Nutritional Analysis: 1 serving equals 118 calories, 6.5 g fat, 29 g carbohydrate, 26.5 g protein
Diabetic Exchanges: 1 vegetable, 2 lean protein

Cherry Corn Muffins

2 cups frozen unsweetened pitted dark sweet cherries

½ cup plus 1 tablespoon granulated sugar, divided

1 cup all-purpose flour

¾ cup yellow cornmeal

1 tablespoon baking powder

¼ teaspoon salt

1 can (14.75 ounces) cream-style corn

¾ cup fat-free liquid egg substitute

⅔ cup fat-free plain Greek yogurt

Preheat oven to 375 degrees.

Place cherries in a microwave-safe bowl and microwave for 1-2 minutes, until completely thawed. Do not drain.

Transfer cherries and any excess liquid to a blender or large food processor. Add 1 tablespoon sugar. Pulse briefly, just until cherries reach a roughly chopped consistency. (Do not puree.) Set aside.

In a large bowl, combine flour, cornmeal, baking powder, salt, and remaining ½ cup sugar. Mix well and set aside.

In a medium bowl, combine cream-style corn, egg substitute, and yogurt. Mix thoroughly.

Add contents of the medium bowl to the large one and stir well. Add cherry mixture and gently stir. Set aside.

Line a 12-cup muffin pan with baking cups and/or spray with nonstick spray. Evenly distribute batter among the 12 cups—cups will be full to the brim.

Bake in the oven until a toothpick inserted into the center of a muffin comes out clean, 25-30 minutes. (FYI: These muffins rise significantly when baked!)

Remove muffins from the pan and allow to cool (on a cooling rack, if you have one).

Note: Combine with 1 serving of the Country Scrambled Eggs

Yield: 12 servings
Nutritional Analysis: 1 serving equals 158 calories, 0.5 g fat, 33 g carbohydrate, 5 g protein
Diabetic Exchanges: 1 starch

Chicken Cheddar Wraps

½ cup (4 ounces) fat-free sour cream

¾ cup chunky salsa

2 tablespoons light mayonnaise

4 (1 pound) boneless skinless chicken breast halves

1 cup (4 ounces) fat-free shredded

cheddar cheese

½ cup thinly sliced fresh mushrooms

2 cups shredded lettuce

6 low-carb, fat-free flour tortillas

Tomato wedges

In a bowl, combine the sour cream, salsa, and mayonnaise. Stir in chicken, cheese, and mushrooms. Divide lettuce between tortillas. Place about ½ cup chicken mixture on each tortilla. Fold sides over the fillings. Garnish with tomato.

Yield: 6 wraps
Nutritional Analysis: 1 wrap equals 167 calories, 3 g fat, 17 g carbohydrate, 18 g protein
Diabetic Exchanges: 1 starch, 2 lean meat, 1 vegetable

Country Scrambled Eggs

12 egg whites, 2 yokes

¾ cup diced fully cooked ham

¾ cup fat-free shredded cheddar cheese

½ cup chopped fresh mushrooms

¼ cup chopped onion

In a bowl, beat eggs. Add ham, cheese, mushrooms, and onion. Lightly coat skillet with cooking spray; add egg mixture. Cook and stir over medium heat until eggs are completely set and cheese is melted.

Yield: 4 servings
Nutritional Analysis: 1 serving equals 134 calories, 6 g fat, 4 g carbohydrate, 16 g protein
Diabetic Exchanges: ½ vegetable, 1 fat, 1.5 lean meats

Creamy Chicken Enchiladas

1 small onion, chopped

1 can (10.75 ounces) reduced-fat, reduced-sodium condensed cream of chicken soup, undiluted

1 can (10 ounces) diced tomatoes and green chilies, undrained

1 cup (8 ounces) fat-free sour cream

1 cup (4 ounces) shredded fat-free cheddar cheese

1 cup (4 ounces) shredded reduced-fat mozzarella cheese

6 low-carb flour tortillas

3 cooked chicken breasts, cubed

In a skillet or saucepan coated with nonstick cooking spray, sauté onion until tender. Remove from heat. Add soup, tomatoes, sour cream, ¾ cup cheddar cheese, and ¾ cup mozzarella cheese; mix well. Divide evenly on each tortilla, top with ½ of a cubed chicken breast. Roll up tightly.

Place seam side down in a 13-inch x 9-inch x 2-inch baking dish coated with nonstick cooking spray. Top with remaining soup mixture; sprinkle with remaining cheeses. Bake uncovered at 350 degrees for 20-25 minutes or until heated through.

Yield: 6 servings
Nutritional Analysis: 1 serving equals 226 calories, 6 g fat, 21 g carbohydrate, 22 g protein
Diabetic Exchanges: 2 lean meat, 1.5 starch, 1 vegetable

Light Turkey Salad Tortillas

12 ounces cooked turkey, shredded or cubed

1 cup (4 ounces) fat-free shredded cheddar cheese

¾ cup finely-chopped celery

½ cup finely-chopped onion

1 can (2.25 ounces) sliced olives, drained

½ cup light mayonnaise

¼ cup picante sauce

6 low-carb flour tortillas (7 inches)

In a bowl, combine the first 7 ingredients, mix well. Evenly divide filling on center on each tortilla. Fold sides and ends over filling, then roll up. Place in a shallow, microwave-safe dish. Cover and microwave on high for 2-3 minutes or until cheese is melted and filling is hot.

Yield: 6 servings
Nutritional Analysis: 1 serving equals 151 calories, 3 g fat, 16 g carbohydrate, 15 g protein
Diabetic Exchanges: ½ starch, 1.5 meat, 1 vegetable

Soft Chicken Tacos

4 (1 pound) boneless skinless chicken breast halves, cubed

1 can (15 ounces) black beans, rinsed and drained

1 cup salsa

1 tablespoon taco seasoning

½ cup fat-free sour cream

6 low-carb, fat-free flour tortillas

Optional Toppings: shredded lettuce, fat-free shredded cheddar cheese, diced tomatoes, and sliced green onions.

In a skillet that has been coated with nonstick cooking spray, cook chicken until juices run clear. Add beans, salsa, and taco seasoning; heat through. Remove from heat and add sour cream. Spoon the chicken mixture down the center of each tortilla. Garnish with toppings of your choice.

Yield: 6 servings
Nutritional Analysis: 1 taco equals 196 calories, 4 g fat, 18 g carbohydrate, 22 g protein
Diabetic Exchanges: 1 starch, 2 lean meat

Recovery Recipes

Blueberry Chicken

4 (1 pound) boneless skinless chicken
    breast halves

1 tablespoon canola oil

¼ cup apricot preserves **or** fruit spread

3 tablespoons Dijon mustard

¼ cup white wine vinegar **or** cider vinegar

1 cup fresh **or** frozen blueberries

In a large skillet over medium heat, cook chicken in oil for about 5 minutes on each side or until lightly browned. Combine preserves and mustard; spoon over chicken. Reduce heat to low; cover and simmer for 20 minutes or until chicken juices run clear.

    With a slotted spoon, remove chicken and keep warm. Add vinegar to skillet; bring to a boil. Reduce heat, simmer uncovered for 3 minutes or until sauce is reduced by one-third, stirring occasionally. Stir in blueberries. Serve rice if desired.

Yield: 4 servings
Nutritional Analysis: 1 serving (prepared with 100% apricot fruit spread) equals 206 calories,
6 g fat, 10 g carbohydrate, 28 g protein
Diabetic Exchanges: 3 lean meat, 1.5 fruit

Chicken Burritos

¼ cup olive oil

¼ cup lime juice

4 garlic cloves, minced

1 tablespoon minced fresh parsley or 1
    teaspoon dried parsley flakes

1 teaspoon ground cumin

1 teaspoon dried oregano

¼ teaspoon pepper

4 (1 pound) boneless skinless chicken
    breast halves

6 low-carb, fat-free flour tortillas

Shredded lettuce, diced tomatoes, and other vegetable condiments of your choice

    In a large resealable plastic bag or shallow glass container, combine the first 7 ingredients. Add chicken and turn to coat. Seal or cover and refrigerate 8 hours or overnight, turning occasionally. Drain and discard marinade. Grill chicken, uncovered, over medium heat for 5-7 minutes on each side or until juices run clear. Cut into thin strips; serve in tortillas or taco shells with desired vegetable condiments.

Yield: 6 servings
Nutritional Analysis: 1 serving equals 201 calories, 5 g fat, 15 g carbohydrate, 24 g protein
Diabetic Exchanges: 3 lean meat, 1 starch, ½ fat

Chicken Veggie Stew

2 pounds boneless skinless chicken breasts, cubed

1 can (14.5 ounces) Italian diced tomatoes, undrained

2 medium potatoes, peeled and cut into ½ inch cubes

6 medium carrots, chopped

4 celery stalks, chopped

1 large onion, chopped

1 medium green pepper, chopped

2 cans (4 ounces **each**) mushrooms, drained

2 low-sodium chicken bouillon cubes

1 teaspoon chili powder

¼ teaspoon pepper

1 tablespoon cornstarch

2 cups water

In a slow cooker, combine the first 11 ingredients. In a small bowl, combine cornstarch and water until smooth. Stir into chicken mixture. Cover and cook on low for 8-10 hours or until vegetables are tender.

Yield: 8 servings
Nutritional Analysis: 1 serving equals 220 calories, 4 g fat, 16 g carbohydrate, 30 g protein
Diabetic Exchanges: 2 vegetable, 3 lean meat, ½ starch

Italian Chicken Cutlets

6 (1.5 pounds) boneless skinless chicken breast halves

1 cup dry bread crumbs

½ cup fat-free Parmesan cheese topping

2 tablespoons wheat germ

1 teaspoon dried basil

½ teaspoon garlic powder

1 cup plain fat-free yogurt

Refrigerated butter-flavored spray

Flatten chicken to ½-inch thickness. In a shallow dish, combine the bread crumbs, Parmesan topping, wheat germ, basil, and garlic powder. Place the yogurt in another shallow dish. Dip chicken in yogurt, then coat with the crumb mixture. Place in a 15-inch x 10-inch x 1-inch baking pan coated with nonstick cooking spray. Spritz chicken with butter-flavored spray. Bake uncovered at 350 degrees for 20-25 minutes or until the juices run clear.

Yield: 6 servings
Nutritional Analysis: 1 serving equals 270 calories, 5 g fat, 15 g carbohydrate, 32 g protein
Diabetic Exchanges: 3 lean meat, 1 starch

Lean and Meaty Spaghetti Sauce

1.5 pounds ground turkey breast

½ pound bulk Italian sausage

1 medium green pepper, chopped

1 medium onion, chopped

8 garlic cloves, minced

3 cans (14.5 ounces **each**) diced tomatoes, drained

2 cans (15 ounces **each**) tomato sauce

2 cans (6 ounces **each**) tomato paste

¼ cup sugar

2 tablespoons Italian seasoning

1 tablespoon dried basil

1 teaspoon salt

½ teaspoon pepper

Hot cooked spaghetti

In a large skillet over medium heat, cook turkey and sausage until no longer pink; drain. Transfer to a 5-quart slower cooker. Stir in green pepper, onion, garlic, tomatoes, tomato sauce, paste, sugar, and seasonings; mix well. Cover and cook on low for 8 hours or until bubbly. Serve over spaghetti.

Yield: 12 servings

Nutritional Analysis: 1 serving (calculated without spaghetti—add macronutrient values for amount of spaghetti served) equals 180 calories, 4 g fat, 12 g carbohydrate, 24 g protein

Diabetic Exchanges: 1 starch, 2 meat, 1 vegetable

Southwest Chicken

4 (1 pound) boneless skinless chicken breast halves

16 ounces picante sauce

2 tablespoons brown sugar

1 tablespoon mustard

Place chicken in a greased shallow 2-quart baking dish. In a small bowl, combine the picante sauce, brown sugar, and mustard; pour over chicken. Bake uncovered at 400 degrees for 30-35 minutes. Serve over rice if desired.

Yield: 4 servings

Nutritional Analysis: 1 serving (calculated without rice) equals 224 calories, 4 g fat, 19 g carbohydrate, 28 g protein

Diabetic Exchanges: 3 lean meat, ½ starch

Spicy White Chili

2 pounds boneless skinless chicken breasts, cubed

1 small onion, chopped

2 cups low-sodium chicken broth

1 can (4 ounces) chopped green chilies

½ teaspoon garlic powder

½ teaspoon dried oregano

½ teaspoon minced fresh cilantro **or** parsley

¼ teaspoon cayenne pepper

1 can (15 ounces) white kidney or cannellini beans, rinsed and drained

In a saucepan coated with nonstick cooking spray, sauté chicken and onion until juices run clear; drain if desired. Stir in broth, chilies, garlic powder, oregano, cilantro, and cayenne. Bring to a boil. Reduce heat; simmer, uncovered, for 30 minutes. Stir in beans; cook 10 minutes longer.

Yield: 8 servings
Nutritional Analysis: 1 serving equals 220 calories, 4 g fat, 14 g carbohydrate, 32 g protein
Diabetic Exchanges: 3.5 lean meat, 1 starch, 1 vegetable

Spinach Chicken Wraps

1 package (10 ounces) fresh spinach

½ cup chopped fresh mushrooms

1 green onion, finely-chopped

1 garlic cloves, minced

1 tablespoon olive oil

2 egg whites, lightly-beaten

¼ cup crumbled feta cheese

¼ cup dry bread crumbs

¼ teaspoon dried rosemary, crushed

4 (1 pound) boneless skinless chicken breast halves

½ teaspoon dried basil

½ teaspoon dried thyme

¼ teaspoon pepper

4 low-carb, fat-free flour tortilla wraps

In a large saucepan, place spinach in a steamer basket over 1 inch of boiling water. Cover and steam for 2-3 minutes or just until wilted. When cool enough to handle, squeeze spinach dry and finely chop. In a nonstick skillet, sauté the mushrooms, onion, and garlic in oil until tender. Add spinach; cook and stir for 2 minutes. Transfer to a bowl. Add egg whites, cheese, and bread crumbs, mix well. Flatten chicken to ¼-inch thickness. Combine basil, thyme, and pepper; rub over one side of chicken. Spread spinach mixture over wraps and roll up. Secure with toothpicks. In a large saucepan, place wraps in a steamer basket over 1 inch of boiling water. Cover and steam for 12-15 minutes or until chicken is no longer pink.

Yield: 4 servings
Nutritional Analysis: 1 serving equals 238 calories, 6 g fat, 16 g carbohydrate, 30 g protein
Diabetic Exchanges: 2 lean meat, 1 vegetable, 1 fat

Anchor Recipes

Artichoke and Olive Tuna Salad Wrap

1 (6 ounces) can chunk light tuna in water, drained and flaked

½ cup chopped canned artichoke hearts

¼ cup chopped olives

3 tablespoons fat-free, plain Greek yogurt

1 teaspoon lemon juice

¼ teaspoon dried oregano

1 whole-grain tortilla

Combine tuna, artichokes, olives, yogurt, lemon juice, and oregano in a medium bowl and mix until moist.

Spoon mixture into tortilla.

Yield: 1 serving
Nutritional Analysis: 1 serving equals 466 calories, 8.5 g fat, 29 g carbohydrate, 55 g protein
Diabetic Exchanges: 3.5 meat/cheese, 1 vegetable, 2 starch

Black Bean, Quinoa, and Sweet Potato Casserole

1 cup quinoa

2 cans seasoned black beans

200 grams raw sweet potato, shredded (can be left out if carbs are an issue)

100 grams (about 4 eggs) egg whites

8 ounces low-fat cheddar cheese, divided

1 cup hot picante sauce or salsa of your choice

1 tablespoon cumin

1 teaspoon chili powder

½ teaspoon garlic powder

1 teaspoon coriander

1 tablespoon cilantro

½ cup onions

1 cup green and jalapeno peppers (to your taste)

Cook quinoa per instructions on box. Cook onion and peppers until tender. Preheat oven to 350 degrees. Mix quinoa, beans, sweet potatoes, ½ cup cheese and seasoning together. Mix egg whites and salsa together. Combine bean mix and salsa mix and put into a casserole dish. Top with ½ cup cheese and bake for approximately 45 minutes (or until set).

Yield: 16 servings
Nutritional Analysis: 1 serving equals 154 calories, 3 g fat, 23.5 g carbohydrate, 10.5 g protein
Diabetic Exchanges: 1 starch, ½ meat/cheese, ½ fat

Garden Tuna Sandwiches

2 cans (6 ounces **each**)
   water-packed tuna, drained

½ cup chopped peeled cucumber

½ shredded carrot

¼ cup finely chopped green onions

½ cup fat-free mayonnaise

¼ cup Dijon mustard

1 tablespoon fat-free sour cream

1 teaspoon lemon juice

¼ teaspoon pepper

8 slices whole wheat bread

4 lettuce leaves

In a bowl, combine the tuna, cucumber, carrot, onions, mayonnaise, mustard, sour cream, lemon juice, and pepper. Spread on four slices of bread; top with lettuce and remaining bread.

Yield: 4 servings
Nutritional Analysis: 1 sandwich equals 236 calories, 4 g fat, 32 g carbohydrate, 18g protein
Diabetic Exchanges: 2 starch, 1.5 lean meat, 1 vegetable

Strawberry Protein Pancakes with Yogurt Filling

Pancake Roll-Ups:

¼ cup low-fat plain Greek yogurt

½ scoop Diet Doc Vanilla Bean protein
   powder

½ teaspoon baking powder

2 egg whites

½ cup regular old-fashioned oats

¼ cup strawberries, chopped

2 tablespoons water

Non-calorie sweetener to taste

Yogurt Filling:

½ cup fat-free plain Greek yogurt

2 tablespoons low-sugar strawberry jam

1-2 packets stevia (or sweetener of
   choice)

Put all of the ingredients for the pancakes in a blender and blend until smooth.

Meanwhile, heat a nonstick griddle (or large nonstick skillet) coated with cooking spray over medium heat. Spoon ½ of the batter (if making 2 large pancakes) or ¼ of the batter (if making 4 smaller pancakes) onto pre-heated griddle. Turn pancakes over when tops are covered with bubbles and edges look cooked. Remove from griddle when both sides are cooked, and place pancakes on a serving plate.

To make the filling, simply mix Greek yogurt with jam and sweetener in a small bowl.

Divide filling between pancakes and roll pancakes up around filling. Place roll-ups on plate seam-side down so they stay rolled, or secure with a toothpick. Serve with strawberries, low-sugar jam, or low-sugar maple syrup if desired.

Yield: 2 large pancakes
Nutritional Analysis: 1 serving (one large pancake) equals 131 calories, 2.5 g fat,
28 g carbohydrate, 15 g protein
Diabetic Exchanges: 1.5 starch, 1 meat/cheese, ½ fat

Vegetarian Burritos

10 egg whites (or equivalent egg substitute)

¼ teaspoon pepper

1 cup salsa

¼ cup chopped onion

1 cup (4 ounces) fat-free shredded cheddar cheese

8 low-carb, fat-free flour tortillas

In a bowl, beat the eggs and pepper. Pour into a skillet that has been coated with nonstick cooking spray. Cook and stir over medium heat until eggs are partially set. Add salsa and onion, cook, and stir until eggs are completely set. Sprinkle with cheese. Spoon about ½ cup down the center of each tortilla; fold ends and sides over filling. Serve immediately.

Yield: 8 servings
Nutritional Analysis: 1 serving equals 146 calories, 2 g fat, 20 g carbohydrate, 12 g protein
Diabetic Exchanges: 1 starch, 1 vegetable, 1 lean meat

Pre-Workout Recipes

Blueberry Pie

¼ cup sugar

Sugar substitute, such as Splenda or Stevia, equivalent to ¼ cup sugar

2 tablespoons cornstarch

¾ cup water

4 cups fresh **or** frozen blueberries, thawed

1 reduced-fat graham cracker crust (9 inches)

Fat-free whipped topping

In a saucepan, combine sugar and cornstarch. Stir in water until smooth. Bring to a boil over medium heat, cook and stir for 2 minutes. Add blueberries. Cook for 3 minutes, stirring occasionally. Pour into crust. Chill. Garnish with whipped topping.

Yield: 8 servings
Nutritional Analysis: 1 piece equals 94 calories, 2 g fat, 17 g carbohydrate, 2 g protein
Diabetic Exchanges: 1 starch, 1 fruit

Cheesy Cornbread Muffins

1 cup canned cream-style corn

⅔ cup all-purpose flour

½ cup yellow cornmeal

½ cup fat-free liquid egg substitute

½ cup fat-free sour cream

½ cup reduced-fat shredded cheddar

cheese

¼ cup chopped scallions

2 tablespoons non-calorie sweetener

1.5 teaspoons baking powder

¼ teaspoon salt

Optional: ¼ teaspoon hot sauce

Preheat oven to 375 degrees.

Combine flour, cornmeal, sweetener, baking powder, and salt in a large bowl. In a separate small bowl, mix together all other ingredients—then add the contents of the small bowl to the large one, and stir until well mixed.

Spray a 12-cup muffin pan with nonstick spray or line it with baking cups. Evenly distribute muffin batter among the cups. Bake in the oven for 15-20 minutes (until muffins are firm and a light golden brown). Allow to cool and then enjoy!

Yield: 12 servings
Nutritional Analysis: 1 serving (one muffin) equals 85 calories, 1.5 g fat,
14 g carbohydrate, 4 g protein
Diabetic Exchanges: ½ starch, ½ fat

Chocolate Mousse

¾ cup skim milk

1 package (1.4 ounces) sugar-free instant chocolate pudding mix

½ cup fat-free sour cream

3 ounces fat-free cream cheese, cubed

½ teaspoon vanilla extract

1 carton (8 ounces) fat-free whipped topping

1 tablespoon chocolate cookie crumbs

In a bowl, whisk milk and pudding mix for 2 minutes (mixture will be very thick). In a mixing bowl, beat the sour cream, cream cheese, and vanilla. Add pudding; mix well. Fold in whipped topping. Spoon into individual dishes. Sprinkle with cookie crumbs. Refrigerate until serving.

Yield: 6 servings
Nutritional Analysis: 1 serving equals 106 calories, 2 g fat, 18 g carbohydrate, 4 g protein
Diabetic Exchanges: 1.5 starch

Double-Stack Fudgy Cheesecake Cupcakes

1 tub (8 ounces) fat-free cream cheese, room temperature

¼ cup fat-free liquid egg substitute

⅓ cup granulated sugar substitute

1 drop vanilla extract

½ of an 18.25-ounce box (about 1.75 cups) moist-style devil's food cake mix

¾ cup club soda

½ cup mini semi-sweet chocolate chips

Preheat oven to 350 degrees. Line a 12-cup muffin pan with foil baking liners.

In a medium bowl, combine cream cheese, egg substitute, sweetener, and vanilla extract.

With an electric mixer set to medium speed, beat until smooth. In a large bowl, whisk cake mix with soda until smooth.

Evenly distribute cake mixture among the lined cups of the muffin pan. Smooth out the mixture with the back of a spoon.

Evenly distribute cream-cheese mixture among the cups. Sprinkle with chocolate chips.

Bake until a toothpick inserted into the center of a cupcake comes out mostly clean, 24-26 minutes. (Make sure the chocolate cake layer is cooked through.)

Allow to cool completely. (Refrigerate leftovers.)

Yield: 12 servings
Nutritional Analysis: 1 serving (one cupcake) equals 153 calories, 4.5 g fat, 25 g carbohydrate, 4.5 g protein
Diabetic Exchanges: 1 starch, 1 fat

Light Carrot Cake

Sugar substitute equivalent to ¼ cup
    sugar

1 tablespoon canola oil

½ cup sugar-free apple sauce

⅓ cup orange juice concentrate

3 egg whites

1 cup all-purpose flour

1 teaspoon baking powder

1 teaspoon ground cinnamon

½ teaspoon ground allspice

¼ teaspoon baking soda

1 cup grated carrots

2 teaspoons confectioners' sugar

In a mixing bowl, combine the first 5 ingredients; beat for 30 seconds. Combine flour, baking powder, cinnamon, allspice, and baking soda; add to the orange juice mixture and mix well. Stir in carrots. Pour into an 8-inch square baking pan that has been coated with nonstick cooking spray. Bake at 350 degrees for 30 minutes or until a toothpick inserted near the center comes out clean. Cool; dust with confectioners' sugar.

Yield: 9 servings
Nutritional Analysis: 1 serving equals 147 calories, 3 g fat, 27 g carbohydrate, 3 g protein
Diabetic Exchanges: 2 starch, ½ fat

No-Bake Chocolate Cheesecake

¾ cup (about 12 squares) reduced-fat
    graham cracker crumbs

2 tablespoons canola oil-based butter

1 envelope unflavored gelatin

1 cup cold water

4 squares (1 ounce **each**) semisweet
    chocolate, coarsely-chopped

4 packages (8 ounces **each**) fat-free

cream cheese

Sugar substitute equivalent to 1 cup sugar

¼ cup sugar

¼ cup baking cocoa

2 teaspoons vanilla extract

Topping:

2 cups fresh raspberries

1 ounce white candy coating

In a bowl, combine cracker crumbs and butter; press onto the bottom of a 9-inch springform pan. Bake at 375 degrees for 8-10 minutes or until lightly browning. Cool on a wire rack.

    For filling, in a small saucepan, sprinkle gelatin over cold water; let stand for 1 minute. Heat over low heat, stirring until gelatin is completely dissolved. Add the semisweet chocolate; stir until melted. In a mixing bowl, beat the cream cheese, sugar substitute, and sugar until smooth. Gradually add the chocolate mixture and cocoa. Beat in vanilla. Pour into crust; refrigerate for 2-3 hours or until firm. Arrange raspberries on top of cheesecake. In a heavy saucepan or microwave, melt white candy coating; stir until smooth. Drizzle or pipe over berries. Carefully run a knife around edge of pan to loosen. Remove sides of pan.

Yield: 12 servings
Nutritional Analysis: 1 slice equals 158 calories, 6 g fat, 27 g carbohydrate, 9 g protein
Diabetic Exchanges: 2 starch, 1 lean meat, 1 fat

Oat Waffles

1 cup all-purpose flour

1 cup oat flour

4 teaspoons baking powder

3 egg whites

1.75 cups skim milk

2 tablespoons canola oil

1 teaspoon vanilla extract

In a bowl, combine the first 3 ingredients. Combine the egg whites, milk, oil, and vanilla; stir into dry ingredients just until combined. Pour ½ cup batter at a time into a preheated waffle iron; bake until golden brown.

Yield: 8 waffles
Nutritional Analysis: 1 waffle equals 147 calories, 3 g fat, 24 g carbohydrate, 6 g protein
Diabetic Exchanges: 1.5 starch

Pear Squares

1 ½ pounds pears, sliced

3 tablespoon all-purpose flour

¼ cup unsweetened apple juice concentrate

¾ cup reduced-fat graham cracker crumbs (about 10 squares)

½ teaspoon ground cinnamon

Dash ground nutmeg

2 tablespoons canola oil-based stick butter

½ cup fat-free whipped topping

Optional: additional ground cinnamon

In a bowl, toss the pears, 1 tablespoon flour, and apple juice concentrate. Spoon into an 8-inch square baking dish coated with nonstick cooking spray.

In a bowl, combine the crumbs, cinnamon, nutmeg, and remaining flour. Cut in butter until mixture resembles coarse crumbs. Sprinkle over pears.

Bake at 375 degrees for 30 minutes or until pears are tender and topping is lightly browned. Serve warm or chilled. Cut into squares; top with whipped topping and cinnamon.

Yield: 9 servings
Nutritional Analysis: 1 serving equals 128 calories, 4 g fat, 22 g carbohydrate, 1 g protein
Diabetic Exchanges: 1 starch, ½ fruit, ½ fat

Post-Workout Recipes

Asian Turkey Tenderloin

20 ounces turkey breast tenderloins

3 tablespoons brown sugar, divided

8 teaspoons reduced-sodium soy sauce, divided

2 tablespoons fresh gingerroot or 1.5

teaspoons ground ginger

6 garlic cloves, minced

½ teaspoon black pepper

1 tablespoon cornstarch

1 cup reduced-sodium chicken broth

Place turkey in a shallow 3-quart baking dish coated with cooking spray. In a small bowl, combine 2 tablespoons brown sugar, 6 teaspoons soy sauce, ginger, garlic and pepper. Set half aside; sprinkle remaining mixture over turkey.

Bake, uncovered, at 375 degrees for 25-30 minutes or until a meat thermometer reads 170 degrees. Let stand for 5 minutes before slicing.

Meanwhile, in a small saucepan, combine the cornstarch and broth until smooth. Stir inreserved soy sauce mixture and remaining brown sugar and soy sauce. Bring to a boil; cook and stir for 2 minutes or until thickened. Serve with turkey.

Yield: 4 servings
Nutritional Analysis: 1 serving (5 ounces turkey with about 2 tablespoons sauce)
equals 212 calories, 2 g fat, 14 g carbohydrate, 35 g protein
Diabetic Exchanges: 5 lean meat, 1 starch

Cajun Salmon Steaks

2 (6 ounces, 1 inch thick) salmon steaks

½ teaspoon Worcestershire sauce

½ teaspoon lemon juice

½ teaspoon Cajun **or** Creole seasoning

½ cup diced green pepper

½ cup diced red pepper

Place the salmon in an ungreased 8-inch square microwave-safe dish. Rub with Worcestershire sauce and lemon juice; sprinkle with Cajun seasoning. Sprinkle peppers on top. Cover and microwave on high for 5-6 minutes, turning once, or until fish flakes easily with a fork. Let stand, covered, for 1 minute.

Yield: 2 servings
Nutritional Analysis: 1 serving equals 268 calories, 12 g fat, 4 g carbohydrate, 36 g protein
Diabetic Exchanges: 3 lean meat, 1 vegetable, 1 fat

Cheese Omelet

4 egg whites

¼ teaspoon onion powder

¼ teaspoon dried basil

¼ teaspoon dried parsley flakes

¼ teaspoon celery seed

¼ cup fat-free shredded cheddar cheese

In a bowl, beat egg whites and seasonings. Lightly coat skillet with cooking spray. Add egg mixture; cook over medium heat. As eggs set, lift edges, letting uncooked portion flow underneath. When eggs are completely set, remove from the heat. Place cheese over half of the eggs. Fold in half and serve.

Yield: 1 serving
Nutritional Analysis: 1 serving equals 118 calories, 2 g fat, 6 g carbohydrate, 19 g protein
Diabetic Exchanges: 1 vegetable, 2 lean protein

Chili Chicken Breasts

1 teaspoon chili powder

½ teaspoon ground cumin

¼ teaspoon garlic powder

¼ teaspoon cayenne pepper

4 (1 pound) boneless skinless chicken breast halves

1 teaspoon canola oil

¼ cup chopped green onions

1 jalapeno pepper, seeded and finely-chopped

1 garlic clove, minced

1 can (14.5 ounces) diced tomatoes, undrained

1 teaspoon cornstarch

2 teaspoons water

Combine the first 4 ingredients, rub over chicken. In a nonstick skillet, brown chicken in oil on both sides. Add onions, jalapeno, and garlic; sauté for 1 minute. Add tomatoes; bring to a boil. Reduce heat; cover and simmer for 15-20 minutes. Remove chicken and keep warm. In a small bowl, combine cornstarch and water until smooth; stir in tomato mixture. Bring to a boil; cook and stir for 1 minute or until slightly thickened. Serve over chicken.

Yield: 4 servings
Nutritional Analysis: 1 serving equals 164 calories, 4 g fat, 4 g carbohydrate, 28 g protein
Diabetic Exchanges: 3 lean meat, 1 vegetable

Cilantro Lime Cod

4 (2 pounds) cod fillets

¼ teaspoon pepper

1 tablespoon dried minced onion

1 garlic clove, minced

1 tablespoon olive oil

1 teaspoon ground cumin

¼ cup minced fresh cilantro or parsley

2 limes, thinly-sliced

1 tablespoon canola oil-based butter

Place each fillet on a 15-inch x 12-inch piece of heavy-duty foil. Sprinkle with pepper. In a small saucepan, sauté onion and garlic in oil; stir in cumin. Spoon over fillets; spinkle with cilantro. Place lime slices over each; drizzle with butter. Fold foil around fish and seal tightly. Place on a baking sheet. Bake at 375 degrees for 35-40 minutes or until fish flakes easily with a fork.

Yield: 8 servings
Nutritional Analysis: 1 serving equals 209 calories, 6 g fat, 3 g carbohydrate, 28 g protein
Diabetic Exchanges: 2 very lean meat, ½ fat

Country Scrambled Eggs

12 egg whites, 2 yolks

¾ cup diced fully cooked ham

¾ cup fat-free shredded cheddar cheese

½ cup chopped fresh mushrooms

¼ cup chopped onion

In a bowl, beat eggs. Add ham, cheese, mushrooms, and onion. Lightly coat skillet with cooking spray; add egg mixture. Cook and stir over medium heat until eggs are completely set and cheese is melted.

Yield: 4 servings
Nutritional Analysis: 1 serving equals 134 calories, 6 g fat, 4 g carbohydrate, 16 g protein
Diabetic Exchanges: ½ vegetable, 1 fat, 1.5 lean meats

Creamed Mushroom Turkey

1 (3 pounds) boneless turkey breast, halved

1 tablespoon canola oil-based butter, melted

2 tablespoons dried parsley flakes

½ teaspoon dried tarragon

½ teaspoon salt

¼ teaspoon pepper

1 jar (4.5 ounces) sliced mushrooms, drained **or** 1 cup sliced fresh mushrooms

½ cup chicken broth

2 tablespoons cornstarch

¼ cup cold water

Place the turkey in a slow cooker. Brush with butter. Sprinkle with parsley, tarragon, salt, and pepper. Top with mushrooms. Pour broth over all. Cover and cook on low for 7-8 hours. Remove turkey and keep warm. Skim fat from cooking juices. In a saucepan, combine cornstarch and water until smooth. Gradually add cooking juices. Bring to a boil; cook and stir for 2 minutes or until thickened. Serve over the turkey.

Yield: 12 servings
Nutritional Analysis: 1 serving equals 191 calories, 7 g fat, 4 g carbohydrate, 28 g protein
Diabetic Exchanges: 3 lean meat, ½ vegetable

Creamy Pea Salad

2 medium carrots, chopped

1 package (16 ounces) frozen peas

1 celery rib, thinly-sliced

¼ cup cubed reduced-fat mozzarella
cheese

2 green onions, thinly-sliced

2 tablespoons buttermilk

2 tablespoons plain nonfat yogurt

1 teaspoon fat-free mayonnaise

½ teaspoon cider or red wine vinegar

½ teaspoon dried basil

¼ teaspoon pepper

In a saucepan, cook carrots in a small amount of boiling water for 2 minutes. Add peas; cook 5 minutes longer. Drain; rinse in cold water and drain again. Place in a bowl; add celery, cheese, and onions. Combine remaining ingredients; pour over pea mixture and toss to coat. Cover and refrigerate for at least 1 hour.

Yield: 5 servings
Nutritional Analysis: 1 (¾ cup) serving equals 103 calories, 3 g fat, 15 g carbohydrate, 4 g protein
Diabetic Exchanges: 1 vegetable, ½ starch

Curry Chicken Breasts

4 (1 pound) boneless skinless chicken
breast halves

1 tablespoon canola oil

¼ cup Worcestershire sauce

2 tablespoons chili sauce

2 teaspoons curry powder

1 teaspoon garlic powder

¼ teaspoon hot pepper sauce

¼ cup chopped onion

In a large skillet, brown chicken on both sides in oil. In a bowl, combine the Worcestershire sauce, chili sauce, curry powder, garlic powder, and hot pepper sauce. Pour over chicken. Add onion. Reduce heat; cover and simmer for 9-11 minutes.

Yield: 4 servings
Nutritional Analysis: 1 serving equals 186 calories, 6 g fat, 4 g carbohydrate, 28 g protein
Diabetic Exchanges: 3 lean meat, 1 vegetable

Dill Salmon

1 (1 pound) salmon fillet

1.5 teaspoons dill weed

½ cup fat-free plain yogurt

½ teaspoon brown sugar

½ teaspoon salt-free seasoning blend

Place the salmon in a 13-inch x 9-inch x 2-inch baking dish coated with nonstick cooking spray and sprinkle with ½ teaspoon dill. Cover and bake at 375 degrees for 20-25 minutes or until the fish flakes easily with a fork. In a small saucepan, combine the yogurt, sugar, seasoning blend, and remaining dill. Cook and stir over low heat until heated through.

Yield: 4 servings
Nutritional Analysis: 1 serving equals 227 calories, 12 g fat, 3 g carbohydrate, 24 g protein
Diabetic Exchanges: 2.5 lean meat, 2 fat

Dilly Scrambled Eggs

6 egg whites, 2 yolks

¼ cup skim milk

Dash pepper

1 teaspoon snipped fresh dill **or** ¼ teaspoon dill weed

In a bowl, beat the eggs, milk, and pepper. Lightly coat skillet with cooking spray; add egg mixture. Cook and stir gently over medium heat until eggs are almost set. Sprinkle with cheese and dill; cook until eggs are completely set and cheese is melted.

Yield: 2 servings
Nutritional Analysis: 1 serving equals 139 calories, 7 g fat, 3 g carbohydrate, 16 g protein
Diabetic Exchanges: 1 fat, 2 lean protein

Garlic Chicken

½ cup dry bread crumbs

¼ cup reduced-fat grated Parmesan cheese

2 tablespoons fresh parsley, minced

¼ teaspoon pepper

¼ cup skim milk

6 (1.5 pounds) boneless skinless chicken breast halves

¼ cup canola oil-based butter

2 garlic cloves, minced

2 tablespoons lemon juice

Pinch paprika

In a large resealable plastic bag, combine the first 5 ingredients. Place milk in a shallow bowl. Dip chicken in milk, and then shake in the crumb mixture. Place in a greased 13-inch x 9-inch x 2-inch baking dish. Combine the butter, garlic, and lemon juice; drizzle over the chicken. Sprinkle with paprika. Bake uncovered at 350 degrees for 25-30 minutes.

Yield: 6 servings
Nutritional Analysis: 1 serving equals 172 calories, 6 g fat, 4 g carbohydrate, 30 g protein
Diabetic Exchanges: 3 lean meat, 1 fat, ½ starch

Herbed Lime Chicken

1 bottle (16 ounces) fat-free Italian salad
   dressing

½ cup lime juice

1 lime, halved and sliced

3 garlic cloves, minced

1 teaspoon dried thyme

8 (2 pounds) boneless skinless
   chicken breast halves

In a bowl, combine the first 5 ingredients. Remove ½ cup for basting; cover and refrigerate. Pour remaining marinade into a large resealable plastic bag; add chicken. Seal bag and turn to coat; refrigerate for 8-10 hours. Drain and discard marinade. Grill chicken, uncovered, over medium heat for 5 minutes. Turn chicken; baste with the reserved marinade. Grill 5-7 minutes longer, basting occasionally.

Yield: 8 servings

Nutritional Analysis: 1 serving equals 172 calories, 4 g fat, 6 g carbohydrate, 28 g protein

Diabetic Exchanges: 3 lean meat

Italian Orange Roughy Fillets

1 pound orange roughy fillets

½ cup tomato juice

1 tablespoon white vinegar

1 envelope Italian salad dressing mix

¼ cup chopped green onions

¼ cup chopped green pepper

Place fish fillets in a shallow 2-quart glass baking dish, positioning the thickest portion of fish toward the outside edges. Combine tomato juice, vinegar, and salad dressing mix; pour over fish. Cover and refrigerate for 30 minutes.

   Sprinkle with onions and green pepper. Cover and bake at 400 for 15 minutes or until fish flakes easily with a fork. Let stand covered for 2 minutes.

Yield: 4 servings

Nutritional Analysis: 1 serving equals 122 calories, 2 g fat, 5 g carbohydrate, 21 g protein

Diabetic Exchanges: 2 very lean meat

Italian-Tomato Chicken

4 (1 pound) boneless skinless chicken
   breast halves

½ cup fat-free Italian salad dressing

8 tomato slices, ¼ inch thick

4 teaspoons seasoned bread crumbs

1 teaspoon minced fresh basil or ¼
   teaspoon dried basil

1 tablespoon grated, reduced-fat
   Parmesan cheese

Place chicken in a shallow bowl; pour ¼ cup dressing over chicken. Cover and refrigerate for 2 hours. Transfer chicken to a shallow baking dish; discard marinade. Drizzle with remaining dressing. Cover and bake at 400 degrees for 10 minutes. Top each chicken breast with tomato slices, crumbs, basil, and cheese. Cover and bake for 10 minutes. Uncover and bake 10-15 minutes longer or until chicken juices run clear.

Yield: 4 servings

Nutritional Analysis: 1 serving equals 164 calories, 4 g fat, 8 g carbohydrate, 28 g protein

Diabetic Exchanges: 3 lean meat, ½ starch

Lean Swedish Meatballs

2 egg whites, lightly-beaten

¼ cup ketchup

¾ cup dry bread crumbs

2 tablespoons dried parsley flakes

2 tablespoons Worcestershire sauce

1 teaspoon onion powder

1 teaspoon garlic powder

1 teaspoon pepper

½ teaspoon salt

½ teaspoon chili powder

3 pounds ground turkey breast

Additional ingredients:

2 envelopes brown gravy mix

½ cup fat-free sour cream

In a bowl, combine the first 10 ingredients. Crumble meat over mixture and mix well. Shape into 1-inch balls (about 6 dozen). Combine brown gravy mix and sour cream and coat meat balls. Place in a single layer in ungreased 15-inch x 10-inch x 1-inch baking pans. Bake at 400 degrees for 20 minutes or until no longer pink, turning often. Remove from the oven; stir in sour cream. Cool.

Yield: 75 meatballs per batch, 15 servings
Nutritional Analysis: 5 Swedish meatballs equal 223 calories, 7 g fat, 8 g carbohydrate, 32 g protein
Diabetic Exchanges: 4 lean meat, ½ starch

Lemon Baked Salmon

1 salmon fillet (2 pounds)

2 tablespoons canola oil-based butter

¼ cup white wine

2 tablespoons lemon juice

½ teaspoon pepper

½ teaspoon dried tarragon

Sliced lemon

Pat salmon dry. Place in a greased 13-inch x 9-inch x 2-inch baking dish. Brush with butter. Combine remaining ingredients; pour over salmon. Top salmon with lemon slices. Bake uncovered at 425 degrees for 20-25 minutes or until fish flakes easily with a fork.

Yield: 8 servings
Nutritional Analysis: 1 (4-ounce) serving equals 192 calories, 8 g fat, 2 g carbohydrate, 28 g protein
Diabetic Exchanges: 4 lean meat, 1 fat

Lemon Chicken

½ cup water

¼ cup lemon juice

2 tablespoons dried minced onion

1 tablespoon dried parsley flakes

1 tablespoon Worcestershire sauce

1 garlic clove, minced

1 teaspoon dill seed

½ teaspoon curry powder

½ teaspoon pepper

8 (2 pounds) boneless skinless chicken breast halves, cut up

In a large resealable bag or shallow glass container, combine the first 9 ingredients. Add chicken and turn to coat. Seal or cover and refrigerate for 4-6 hours. Drain and discard marinade. Grill chicken, covered, over low heat for 50-60 minutes or until juices run clear, turning several times.

Yield: 8 servings
Nutritional Analysis: 1 serving equals 156 calories, 4 g fat, 2 g carbohydrates, 28 g protein
Diabetic Exchanges: 3 lean meat

Lemon Fish

1 pound whitefish or sole fillets

¼ cup lemon juice

1 teaspoon olive oil

2 teaspoons salt-free lemon-pepper seasoning

1 small onion, thinly sliced

1 teaspoon dried parsley flakes

Cut fish into serving-size pieces. Place in an ungreased 11-inch x 7-inch x 2-inch baking dish. Drizzle with lemon juice and oil; sprinkle with lemon pepper. Arrange onion over fish; sprinkle with parsley. Cover and let stand for 5 minutes. Bake at 350 degrees for 20 minutes or until fish flakes easily with a fork.

Yield: 4 servings
Nutritional Analysis: 1 serving equals 156 calories, 6 g fat, 2 g carbohydrate, 28 g protein
Diabetic Exchanges: 3 very lean meat

Light Spinach Quiche

3 ounces fat-free cream cheese

1 cup skim milk

8 egg whites

¼ teaspoon pepper

3 cups (12 ounces) shredded fat-free cheddar cheese

1 package (10 ounces) frozen chopped spinach, thawed and squeezed dry

1 cup frozen chopped broccoli, thawed and well-drained

1 small onion, finely-chopped

5 fresh mushrooms, sliced

In a small mixing bowl, beat cream cheese. Add milk, egg whites, and pepper; beat until smooth. Stir in remaining ingredients. Transfer to a 10-inch quiche pan coated with nonstick cooking spray. Bake at 350 degrees for 45-50 minutes or until a knife inserted near the center comes out clean.

Yield: 8 servings
Nutritional Analysis: 1 serving equals 122 calories, 2 g fat, 8 g carbohydrate, 18 g protein
Diabetic Exchanges: 1 starch, 1 meat

Mini Turkey Loaves

4 egg whites

½ cup fat-free plain yogurt

1 can (6 ounces) tomato paste

2 tablespoons Worcestershire sauce

½ cup quick-cooking oats

1 small onion, chopped

2 tablespoons dried parsley flakes

1 teaspoon salt

½ teaspoon garlic powder

½ teaspoon pepper

2 pounds ground turkey breast

½ cup low-carb ketchup

In a large bowl, combine the first 10 ingredients. Crumble turkey over mixture and mix well. Shape into eight loaves. Place on a rack coated with nonstick cooking spray in a shallow baking pan. Bake uncovered at 350 degrees for 30 minutes. Spoon ketchup over the loaves. Bake 15 minutes longer.

Yield: 8 servings
Nutritional Analysis: 1 serving equals 172 calories, 4 g fat, 2 g carbohydrates, 30 g protein
Diabetic Exchanges: 3 lean meat, 1 starch, ½ fat

Mushroom Spinach Tart

2 tablespoons seasoned bread crumbs

½ pound fresh mushrooms, sliced

½ cup chopped onion

1 tablespoon olive oil

1 package (10 ounces) frozen chopped spinach, thawed and squeezed dry

1 cup skim milk

1 cup egg substitute

¼ teaspoon salt

¼ teaspoon pepper

1 cup shredded reduced-fat Mexican cheese

½ cup grated reduced-fat Parmesan cheese

Coat a 9-inch pie plate with nonstick cooking spray. Sprinkle bottom and sides with bread crumbs; shake out the excess. Set plate aside. In a nonstick skillet, sauté mushrooms and onion in oil for 12-14 minutes or until all of the liquid has evaporated. Remove from the heat; stir in spinach.

In a bowl, combine the milk, egg substitute, salt, and pepper. Stir in the spinach mixture, 1 cup Mexican cheese blend and Parmesan cheese. Pour into prepared pie plate. Bake at 350 degrees for 35-40 minutes or until a knife inserted near the center comes out clean. Sprinkle remaining cheese around edge of tart. Let stand for 5 minutes before slicing.

Yield: 8 servings
Nutritional Analysis: 1 piece equals 176 calories, 8 g fat, 10 g carbohydrate, 16 g protein
Diabetic Exchanges: 2 lean meat, 1 vegetable, 1 fat, ½ starch

Mushroom Turkey Burger

2 pounds ground turkey breast

1 can (4 ounces) mushroom stems and pieces, drained

¼ cup egg substitute

½ cup chopped onion

¼ cup ketchup

1 teaspoon Italian seasoning

¼ teaspoon pepper

¼ teaspoon Worcestershire sauce

In a bowl, combine all ingredients. Divide into 8 patties and grill, covered, over medium heat until meat is no longer pink, turning once.

Yield: 8 servings
Nutritional Analysis: 1 serving equals 186 calories, 6 g fat, 4 g carbohydrate, 29 g protein
Diabetic Exchanges: 3 lean meat, 1 vegetable

Oriental Sesame Chicken

1 pound boneless skinless chicken breasts, cubed

1 tablespoon canola oil

¼ cup light soy sauce

¼ cup sesame seeds

1 large onion, sliced

2 jars (4.5 ounces **each**) sliced mushrooms, drained, **or** 2 cups sliced fresh mushrooms

In a large skillet, cook chicken in oil until no longer pink. Stir in the soy sauce and sesame seeds. Cook and stir over medium heat for 5 minutes. Remove chicken with a slotted spoon; set aside and keep warm. In the same skillet, sauté onion and mushrooms until onion is tender. Return chicken to pan; heat through.

Yield: 4 servings
Nutritional Analysis: 1 serving equals 212 calories, 8 g fat, 6 g carbohydrate, 29 g protein
Diabetic Exchange: 4 very lean meat, 1 fat, 1 vegetable

Parmesan Chicken

½ cup dry bread crumbs

½ cup grated reduced-fat Parmesan cheese

2 tablespoons minced fresh parsley

1 garlic clove, minced

¼ teaspoon pepper

4 egg whites

8 (2 pounds) boneless skinless chicken breast halves

½ cup sliced almonds

Butter-flavored cooking spray

In a shallow bowl, combine the first 5 ingredients. In another shallow bowl, beat the egg whites. Dip chicken in egg whites, then coat with crumb mixture. Place in a 13-inch x 9-inch x 2-inch baking dish coated with nonstick cooking spray.

Sprinkle almonds over chicken. Spritz lightly with butter-flavored spray. Bake uncovered at 350 degrees for 30 minutes.

Yield: 8 servings
Nutritional Analysis: 1 serving equals 216 calories, 8 g fat, 6 g carbohydrate, 30 g protein
Diabetic Exchanges: 3 lean meat, ½ starch

Pumpkin Cupcakes with Protein Frosting

3 scoops Diet Doc Vanilla Bean protein powder

9 egg whites

¾ cup canned pumpkin

6 tablespoons ground flaxseed

8 packets or 2 teaspoons Stevia

3 tablespoons unsweetened dark chocolate cocoa powder

2 teaspoons baking powder

Frosting:

1 cup Diet Doc Vanilla Bean protein powder

2 teaspoons cinnamon, to taste

2 packets or ½ teaspoon stevia

Preheat oven to 350 degrees. Line a 12-cup muffin tin with paper liners. Combine all ingredients in a mixing bowl. Use an electric or hand mixer to blend thoroughly together.

Divide mixture into lined muffin tins. Bake for about 15 minutes or until cooked fully through. To test, insert a toothpick into one and if the pick comes out clean, then it is ready. Remove from the oven.

To make frosting, mix all ingredients in a small bowl. Add water slowly and stir until smooth. Spread evenly on top of each cupcake.

Yield: 12 servings
Nutritional Analysis: 1 serving (one cupcake) equals 150 calories, 2 g fat, 12 g carbohydrate, 21 g protein
Diabetic Exchanges: 1 lean protein, ½ starch

Orange Roughy Primavera

1 tablespoon canola oil-based butter

4 (4 ounces each) orange roughy fillets, thawed

2 tablespoons lemon juice

Dash pepper

1 garlic clove, minced

1 tablespoon olive oil

1 cup broccoli florets

1 cup cauliflowerets

1 cup julienned carrots

1 cup sliced fresh mushrooms

½ cup sliced celery

¼ teaspoon dried basil

¼ teaspoon salt

¼ cup reduced-fat, grated Parmesan cheese

Place butter in a 13-inch x 9-inch x 2-inch baking dish; add fish and turn to coat. Sprinkle with lemon juice and pepper. Bake uncovered at 450 degrees for 5 minutes.

Meanwhile, in a large skillet over medium heat, sauté garlic in oil, add the next 7 ingredients, stir-fry until vegetables are crisp-tender—about 2-3 minutes. Spoon over the fish; sprinkle with cheese. Bake uncovered at 450 degrees for 3-5 minutes or until fish flakes easily with a fork.

Yield: 4 servings
Nutritional Analysis: 1 serving equals 215 calories, 7 g fat, 10 g carbohydrate, 28 g protein
Diabetic Exchanges: 3 very lean meat, 1.5 vegetable, 1 fat

Pork Tenderloin with Sugar Snap Peas

1 pound pork tenderloin, cut into ¼-inch slices

2 garlic cloves, minced

2 teaspoons canola oil

10 ounces fresh or frozen sugar snap peas

3 tablespoons reduced-sodium soy sauce

2 tablespoons white wine vinegar or white vinegar

1 tablespoon molasses

¾ teaspoon ground ginger or 1 tablespoon fresh gingerroot, minced

¼ teaspoon crushed red pepper flakes

In a nonstick skillet, stir-fry pork and garlic in hot oil for 6 minutes or until meat in no longer pink. Remove from skillet. In same pan, cook the peas in soy sauce, vinegar, molasses, ginger and red pepper flakes for 4 minutes or until peas are crisp-tender.

Return pork to pan; cook for 3 minutes or until glazed. Serve warm.

Yield: 4 servings
Nutritional Analysis: 1 serving (1 cup) equals 226 calories, 6 g fat, 10 g carbohydrate, 27 g protein
Diabetic Exchanges: 3 lean meat, 1 vegetable, ½ starch

Shrimp and Veggie Stir-Fry

1.5 pounds medium uncooked shrimp, peeled and deveined

½ teaspoon salt

¼ teaspoon pepper

2 tablespoons canola oil

1 cup fresh broccoli florets

1 cup sweet red pepper, julienned

4 tablespoons reduced-sodium chicken broth, divided

1 cup sliced fresh mushrooms

1.5 cups fresh sugar snap peas

¾ cup sliced green onions

3 garlic cloves, minced

Sprinkle shrimp with salt and pepper. In a large nonstick skillet, stir-fry shrimp in hot oil until shrimp turn pink. Remove with a slotted spoon and keep warm.

In the same pan, stir-fry the broccoli and red pepper in 2 tablespoons broth for 5 minutes.

Add mushrooms; stir-fry for 2 minutes. Add the peas, onions, garlic, and remaining broth; stir-fry for 3-4 minutes or until vegetables are crisp-tender. Return shrimp to the pan ; stir-fry for 1-2 minutes or until heated through.

Yield: 4 servings
Nutritional Analysis: 1 serving (1.5 cups) equals 226 calories, 8 g fat, 12 g carbohydrate, 25 g protein
Diabetic Exchanges: 3 lean meat, 2 vegetable

Sirloin with Portabella Mushroom Sauce

1 pound boneless beef sirloin steak (about ¾ inch thick)

1 teaspoon coarse ground pepper

2 teaspoons canola oil

1 ½ cups sliced fresh portabella mushrooms

½ cup beef broth

½ cup dry red wine or additional beef broth

Rub steak with pepper. In a heavy ovenproof skillet over medium-high heat, brown steak in oil for about 4 minutes on each side. Bake uncovered at 450 degrees for 4 minutes or until meat reaches desired doneness (for rare, a meat thermometer should read 140 degrees; medium, 160; well-done, 170). Transfer steak to a warm serving platter. Let stand for 10 minutes.

In the same skillet, cook mushrooms over medium heat until golden brown. Add broth and wine or additional broth. Bring to a boil; cook until the liquid is reduced by about half. Thinly slice the steak; top with mushroom sauce.

Yield: 4 servings
Nutritional Analysis: 1 serving (3 ounces cooked beef with ¼ cup mushroom sauce) equals 214 calories, 9 g fat, 1 g carbohydrate, 27 g protein
Diabetic Exchanges: 3 lean meat, ½ fat

Spicy Haddock

2 pounds haddock fillets, thawed

1 can (4 ounces) chopped green chilies

1 tablespoon canola oil

1 tablespoon soy sauce

2 tablespoons Worcestershire sauce

1 teaspoon paprika

½ teaspoon garlic powder

½ teaspoon chili powder

Dash hot pepper sauce

Place fillets in a 13-inch x 9-inch x 2-inch baking dish that has been coated with nonstick cooking spray. Combine remaining ingredients; spoon over fish. Bake uncovered at 350 degrees for 20-25 minutes or until fish flakes easily with a fork.

Yield: 8 servings
Nutritional Analysis: 1 (4-ounce) serving equals 155 calories, 5 g fat, 2 g carbohydrate, 28 g protein
Diabetic Exchanges: 3 very lean meat, ½ vegetable

Spinach Egg Bake

1 cup seasoned bread crumbs

2 packages (10 ounces **each**) frozen chopped spinach, thawed and squeezed dry

3 cups (24 ounces) small-curd, fat-free cottage cheese

½ cup grated fat-free Parmesan cheese

8 egg whites, 2 yolks

Sprinkle ¼ cup bread crumbs into a cooking spray-coated 8-inch square baking dish. Bake at 350 degrees for 3-5 minutes or until golden brown.

In a bowl, combine the spinach, cottage cheese, Parmesan cheese, six egg whites, one yolk, and remaining crumbs. Spread over the baked crumbs.

Beat remaining eggs; pour over spinach mixture.

Bake uncovered at 350 degrees for 45 minutes or until a knife inserted near the center comes out clean. Let stand for 5-10 minutes before serving.

Yield: 4 servings
Nutritional Analysis: 1 serving equals 176 calories, 4 g fat, 15 g carbohydrate, 20 g protein
Diabetic Exchanges: 2 lean meat, 1 starch, 1 vegetable, 1 fat

Stuffed Sole

2 tablespoons canola oil-based butter

2 tablespoons lemon juice

½ teaspoon salt

¼ teaspoon pepper

1 package (10 ounces) frozen chopped broccoli, thawed and drained

1 cup cooked rice

1 cup (4 ounces) shredded reduced-fat cheddar cheese

8 (4 ounces **each**) sole **or** whitefish fillets

Paprika

In a small bowl, combine the butter, lemon juice, salt, and pepper. In another bowl, combine the broccoli, rice, cheese, and half of the butter mixture. Spoon ½ cup onto each fillet. Roll up and place seam side down in a baking dish coated with nonstick cooking spray. Pour remaining butter mixture over roll-ups.

Bake uncovered at 350 degrees for 25 minutes or until fish flakes easily with a fork. Baste with pan drippings; sprinkle with paprika.

Yield: 8 servings
Nutritional Analysis: 1 serving equals 231 calories, 7 g fat, 12 g carbohydrate, 30 g protein
Diabetic Exchanges: 3 lean meat, 1 vegetable, ½ starch

Sweet and Spicy Chicken

1 pound boneless skinless chicken
  breasts, cut into ½-inch cubes

3 tablespoons taco seasoning

1 tablespoon canola oil

1 jar (11 ounces) chunky salsa

½ cup sugar-free peach preserves

Coat chicken with taco seasoning. In a skillet, brown chicken in oil. Combine salsa and preserves; stir into skillet. Bring to a boil. Reduce heat; cover and simmer for 2-3 minutes. Serve over rice if desired.

Yield: 4 servings
Nutritional Analysis: 1 serving equals 197 calories, 5 g fat, 10 g carbohydrate, 28 g protein
Diabetic Exchanges: 3 lean meat, 1 fruit, ½ fat

Turkey Tortilla Pie

1 small onion, finely chopped

½ teaspoon garlic powder

1 teaspoon olive oil

1 pound ground turkey breast

2 teaspoons chili powder

1 teaspoon dried oregano

½ teaspoon ground cumin

½ teaspoon cayenne pepper

1 can (15 ounces) black beans, rinsed and
  drained

1 jar (16 ounces) salsa

¾ cup low-sodium chicken broth

8 low-carb, fat-free flour tortillas

½ cup shredded reduced-fat Monterey
  Jack cheese

¼ cup light sour cream

In a skillet, sauté onion and garlic powder in oil until the onion is tender. Add turkey, chili powder, oregano, cumin, and cayenne; cook and stir over medium heat until turkey is no longer pink. Stir in beans. Remove from heat. Combine salsa and broth; spread a thin layer in a 2 ½-quart baking dish coated with nonstick cooking spray. Cut tortillas into 1 inch strips and then into thirds; arrange half over salsa mixture. Top with half of the turkey mixture and half of the remaining salsa mixture. Repeat layers. Sprinkle with cheese. Cover and bake at 350 degrees for 25 minutes or until bubbly. Top individual servings with sour cream.

Yield: 8 servings
Nutritional Analysis: 1 (1 cup) serving equals 270 calories, 6 g fat, 32 g carbohydrate, 22 g protein
Diabetic Exchanges: 2 starch, 2 lean meat, 1 vegetable

Veggie Omelet

¼ cup diced green pepper

¼ cup onion, diced

¼ cup mushrooms, sliced

4 egg whites

Dash pepper

2 tablespoons fat-free shredded cheddar cheese

In an 8-inch skillet, sauté green pepper, onion, and mushrooms in cooking spray until tender. Remove and set aside. In a small bowl, beat egg whites, salt, and pepper. Pour into a skillet. Cook over medium heat; as eggs set, lift edges, letting uncooked portion flow underneath. When the eggs are set, spoon vegetables and cheese over one side; fold omelet over filling. Cover and let stand for 1-2 minutes or until cheese is melted.

Yield: 1 serving
Nutritional Analysis: 1 serving equals 98 calories, 2 g fat, 3 g carbohydrate, 17 g protein
Diabetic Exchanges: 1 vegetable, 2 lean protein

Zesty Cod

1.5 cups water

1 tablespoon lemon juice

2 pounds cod fillets

¼ tsp pepper

1 small onion, finely-chopped

2 large tomatoes, sliced

½ cup chopped green pepper

½ cup seasoned bread crumbs

¼ cup grated, reduced-fat Parmesan cheese

½ teaspoon dried basil

1 tablespoon olive oil

In a bowl, combine the water and lemon juice. Add fish; let sit for 5 minutes. Drain and place in an 11-inch x 7-inch x 2-inch baking dish coated with nonstick cooking spray. Sprinkle with pepper. Layer with onion, tomatoes, and green pepper. Combine the remaining ingredients, sprinkle over top. Bake uncovered at 375 degrees for 20-30 minutes or until fish flakes easily with a fork.

Yield: 8 servings
Nutritional Analysis: 1 serving equals 188 calories, 4 g fat, 10 g carbohydrate, 28 g protein
Diabetic Exchanges: 3 lean meat, 1 starch

Replenish Recipes

Broccoli-Cabbage Slaw

2 cups shredded cabbage

2 cups broccoli florets

1 cup cauliflowerets

1 medium red onion, thinly-sliced

¼ cup reduced-fat mayonnaise

¼ cup fat-free plain yogurt

¼ cup reduced-fat sour cream

¼ cup reduced-fat shredded Parmesan cheese

In a salad bowl, combine the cabbage, broccoli, cauliflower, and onion. In a small bowl, combine the remaining ingredients. Pour over vegetables and toss to coat. Cover and refrigerate until serving.

Yield: 6 servings
Nutritional Analysis: 1 (¾ cup) serving equals 116 calories, 6 g fat, 15 g carbohydrate, 5 g protein
Diabetic Exchanges: 1 vegetable, 1 fat, ½ starch

Broccoli Cheddar Soup

1 (5 cups) large bunch broccoli, coarsely-chopped

2 tablespoons cornstarch

2 cups skim milk

1 cup chicken broth

1 tablespoon canola oil-based butter

¼ teaspoon salt

1/8 teaspoon pepper

1 cup (8 ounces) shredded fat-free cheddar cheese

Dash paprika

In a saucepan, bring 1 inch of water to a boil. Place broccoli in a steamer basket over water. Cover and steam for 5-8 minutes or until crisp-tender. Meanwhile, in another saucepan, combine the cornstarch, milk, and broth until smooth. Bring to a boil, cook, and stir for 2 minutes or until thickened. Stir in the butter, salt, and pepper. Reduce heat. Add cheese and broccoli; heat just until cheese is melted. Sprinkle with paprika.

Yield: 4 servings
Nutritional Analysis: 1 serving equals 123 calories, 3 g fat, 17 g carbohydrate, 7 g protein
Diabetic Exchanges: 2 vegetable, 1 lean meat, 1 fat

Cauliflower Fritters

4 cups steamed cauliflower (roughly-chopped)

2 cloves garlic, crushed

1 cup whole-wheat flour

2 eggs

½ cup Pecorino Romano

¼ cup parsley, finely-chopped

¼ cup hot water

Salt and pepper

¼ cup olive oil

In a large bowl, combine cauliflower, flour, garlic, eggs, grated cheese, parsley, salt and pepper. Add water so that batter becomes slightly denser than pancake batter. On medium-low heat, add 1 tablespoon of oil in a 10-inch skillet coating bottom of the pan. Use a ¼-cup measuring cup to form fritters. You can fit 4 fritters at a time. Cook until golden brown, turn and cook another few minutes. Add a little more oil to the pan and repeat with the remaining batter.

Yield: 24 fritters
Nutritional Analysis: 1 serving (2 fritters) equals 109 calories, 6.5 g fat, 9.5 carbohydrate, 4 g protein
Diabetic Exchanges: ½ vegetable, ½ starch, ½ meat/cheese

Cherry Cream Pie

4 ounces fat-free cream cheese, softened

1.5 cups sugar-free cherry pie filing

2 cups fat-free whipped topping

1 reduced-fat graham cracker crust (9 inches)

In a mixing bowl, beat cream cheese until smooth. Fold in the pie filling and whipped topping until blended. Spoon into crust. Cover and freeze for 8 hours or overnight. Remove from the freezer 15 minutes before serving.

Yield: 8 servings
Nutritional Analysis: 1 piece equals 94 calories, 2 g fat, 15 g carbohydrate, 4 g protein
Diabetic Exchanges: 1 starch, ½ fruit

Creamy Raspberry Pie

1 package (3 ounces) sugar-free raspberry gelatin

½ cup boiling water

1 cup fat-free frozen vanilla yogurt

1 cup fresh **or** frozen unsweetened

raspberries

¼ cup lime juice

2 cups fat-free whipped topping

1 reduced-fat graham cracker crust (9 inches)

Optional: lime slices and additional raspberries and whipped topping

In a bowl, dissolve the gelatin in boiling water. Stir in frozen yogurt until melted. Add raspberries and lime juice. Fold in whipped topping. Spoon into crust. Refrigerate for 3 hours or until firm. Garnish with lime, raspberries, and whipped topping.

Yield: 8 servings
Nutritional Analysis: 1 slice equals 86 calories, 2 g fat, 13 g carbohydrate, 4 g protein
Diabetic Exchanges: 1 starch, ½ fruit

Eggnog Pudding

2 cups skim milk

1 package (3.4 ounces) sugar-free instant
vanilla pudding mix

½ teaspoon ground nutmeg

¼ teaspoon rum extract

Optional: additional nutmeg

In a bowl, combine the first 4 ingredients. Beat for 2 minutes. Spoon into individual dishes. Chill.
Sprinkle with nutmeg if desired.

Yield: 4 servings
Nutritional Analysis: 1 (½ cup) serving equals 101 calories, 1 g fat, 16 g carbohydrate, 7 g protein.
Diabetic Exchanges: 1 starch, ½ lean meat

Extreme Crustless Pumpkin Quiche

1 cup chopped sweet onion

1 cup chopped mushrooms

2 cups chopped spinach leaves

4 wedges Laughing Cow cheese at room

temperature

1 can (15 ounces) pure pumpkin

1 ¼ cups fat-free liquid egg substitute

2 teaspoons chopped garlic

Preheat oven to 350 degrees. Spray a 9-inch pie pan with nonstick spray and set aside.

Bring a large skillet sprayed with nonstick spray to medium-high heat on the stove. Add onion,
and stirring occasionally, cook until softened and slightly browned—about 6 minutes.

Transfer cooked onion to a large bowl and set aside. Remove skillet from heat. If needed,
wash and dry. Spray with nonstick spray and return to medium-high heat. Add mushrooms and,
stirring occasionally, cook until softened and lightly browned, about 4 minutes. Add spinach and
cook until wilted and excess moisture has evaporated, about 2 more minutes.

Transfer mushroom-spinach mixture to the large bowl. Add cheese wedges, breaking them
into pieces as you add them. Mix thoroughly until cheese has melted and is evenly distributed.
Add all remaining ingredients to the bowl and mix well. Evenly transfer mixture to the pie pan.

Bake in the oven until firm and lightly browned on top, about 1 hour.

Allow to slightly cool. Cut into 8 slices.

Yield: 8 servings
Nutritional Analysis: 1 serving equals 67 calories, 1 g fat, 8 g carbohydrate, 6 g protein
Diabetic Exchanges: 1 vegetable, ½ starch, ½ meat/cheese

Italian Mushroom Salad

2 pounds fresh mushrooms, quartered

3 medium tomatoes, cut into wedges

1 cup fat-free Italian salad dressing

1 teaspoon dried parsley flakes

½ teaspoon garlic powder

¼ cup chopped onion

½ teaspoon dried basil

3 cups fresh spinach leaves

4 turkey bacon strips, cooked and chopped

Place mushrooms and tomatoes in a large shallow dish. Combine the next 5 ingredients; drizzle over mushrooms and tomatoes. Cover and refrigerate overnight, stirring once. Line a serving platter or bowl with spinach. Using a slotted spoon, arrange vegetables over spinach. Sprinkle with turkey bacon.

Yield: 8 servings
Nutritional Analysis: 1 (1 cup) serving equals 37 calories, 1 g fat 8 g carbohydrate, 1 g protein
Diabetic Exchanges: 1 vegetable

Lemon Blueberry Cheesecake

1 package (3 ounces) sugar-free lemon gelatin

1 cup boiling water

2 tablespoons canola oil-based butter

1 tablespoon canola oil

1 cup reduced-fat graham cracker crumbs (about 16 squares)

1 carton (24 ounces) fat-free cottage cheese

¼ cup sugar

Sugar substitute equivalent to ¼ cup sugar

Topping:

Sugar substitute equivalent to 2 tablespoons sugar

1.5 teaspoons cornstarch

¼ cup water

1.5 cups fresh or frozen blueberries

1 teaspoon lemon juice

In a bowl, dissolve gelatin in boiling water; cool. Combine butter and oil; add crumbs and blend well. Press onto the bottom of a 9-inch springform pan. Chill. In a blender, process cottage cheese, sugar substitute, and sugar until smooth. While processing, slowly add cooled gelatin. Pour into crust; chill overnight.

For topping, combine sugar substitute and cornstarch in a saucepan; stir in water until smooth. Add 1 cup blueberries. Bring to a boil; cook and stir for 2 minutes or until thickened. Stir in lemon juice; cool slightly. Process in a blender until smooth. Refrigerate until completely cooled. Carefully run a knife around edge of pan to loosen cheesecake; remove sides of pan. Spread the blueberry mixture over the top. Top with remaining blueberries.

Yield: 12 servings
Nutritional Analysis: 1 piece equals 156 calories, 4 g fat, 22 g carbohydrate, 8 g protein
Diabetic Exchanges: 1.5 starch, ½ fruit, ½ fat

Lemon Mousse

¼ cup sugar

Sugar substitute equivalent to ½ cup
  sugar

½ cup cornstarch

3 cups skim milk

⅔ cup lemon juice

1.5 teaspoons grated lemon peel

¼ teaspoon vanilla extract

2 cups fat-free whipped topping

In a saucepan, combine the sugar, sugar substitute, and cornstarch; gradually stir in milk until smooth. Bring to a boil over medium heat, stirring constantly. Cook and stir for 2 minutes or until thickened and bubbly. Remove from the heat. Stir in lemon juice, peel, and vanilla. Set saucepan in ice; stir until mixture reaches room temperature, about 5 minutes. Fold in whipped topping. Spoon into dessert dishes. Refrigerate for at least 1 hour before serving.

Yield: 10 servings
Nutritional Analysis: 1 (½ cup) serving equals 61 calories, 1 g fat, 10 g carbohydrate, 3 g protein
Diabetic Exchanges: 1 starch, 1 fruit

Orange Whip

1 can (11 ounces) mandarin oranges,
  drained

1 cup (8 ounces) fat-free, low-carb vanilla

yogurt

2 tablespoons orange juice concentrate

2 cups fat-free whipped topping

In a bowl, combine the oranges, yogurt, and orange juice concentrate. Fold in the whipped topping. Spoon into serving dishes. Cover and freeze until firm. Remove from the freezer 20 minutes before serving.

Yield: 4 servings
Nutritional Analysis: 1 (¾ cup) serving equals 81 calories, 1 g fat, 15 g carbohydrate, 3 g protein
Diabetic Exchanges: 1 fruit, 1 starch

Peanut Butter Pudding

2 cups skim milk

4 tablespoons reduced-fat creamy peanut butter

1 package (1 ounce) sugar-free instant

vanilla pudding mix

½ cup fat-free whipped topping

4 teaspoons chocolate syrup

In a bowl, whisk the milk and peanut butter until blended. Add pudding mix, whisk for 2 minutes or until slightly thickened. Spoon into dessert dishes. Refrigerate for at least 5 minutes or until set. Just before serving, dollop with shipped topping and drizzle with chocolate syrup.

Yield: 4 servings
Nutritional Analysis: 1 serving equals 172 calories, 8 g fat, 17 g carbohydrate, 8 g protein
Diabetic Exchanges: 1 starch, 1 lean meat, 1 fat

Pumpkin Spice Dip

1 package (8 ounces) fat-free cream cheese

½ cup canned pumpkin

Sugar substitute equivalent to ½ cup sugar

1 teaspoon ground cinnamon

1 teaspoon vanilla extract

1 teaspoon maple flavoring

½ teaspoon pumpkin pie spice

½ teaspoon ground nutmeg

1 carton (8 ounces) fat-free whipped topping

In a large mixing bowl, combine the cream cheese, pumpkin, and sugar substitute; mix well. Beat in the cinnamon, vanilla, maple flavoring, pumpkin pie spice, and nutmeg. Fold in whipped topping. Refrigerate until serving.

Yield: 4 cups
Nutritional Analysis: 1 serving (3 tablespoons) equals 33 calories, 1 g fat, 4 g carbohydrate, 1 g protein
Diabetic Exchanges: ½ starch

Protein Shake Recipes

Banana Nut Blast

½ cup 2% cottage cheese

1 scoop Diet Doc Vanilla Bean protein powder

½ frozen small, very ripe banana

3-5 drops banana extract

2 teaspoons sugar-free vanilla instant pudding mix

1 tablespoon walnuts, chopped

½ teaspoon or 2 packets stevia (or sweetener of choice)

5-10 ice cubes (more or less depending on desired thickness)

Place all ingredients in a blender. Mix until desired consistency is reached, scraping sides if necessary.

Tips: For 11 g fewer carbs, omit frozen fruit and add more banana extract. For 5 g less fat, omit nuts and add walnut extract. For 10g less protein, reduce whey to ⅔ of a scoop.

Yield: 1 serving
Nutritional Analysis: 1 serving equals 366 calories, 10 g fat, 24 g carbohydrate, 45 g protein
Diabetic Exchanges: 2 protein, 1 cheese, 1 fat, ½ fruit

Blueberry Bliss

½ cup frozen blueberries

1 scoop Diet Doc Vanilla Bean protein powder

½ cup fat-free plain Greek yogurt

½ cup unsweetened almond milk

4 packets or 1 teaspoon stevia (or sweetener of choice)

5-10 ice cubes (more or less depending on desired thickness)

Place all ingredients in a blender. Mix until desired consistency is reached, scraping sides if necessary.

Yield: 1 serving
Nutritional Analysis: 1 serving equals 298 calories, 4 g fat, 23 g carbohydrate, 42.5 g protein
Diabetic Exchanges: 2 protein, 1 dairy, 1 fat, ½ fruit

Cake Batter

½ cup low-fat cottage cheese

1 scoop Diet Doc Vanilla Bean protein powder

3-5 drops butter extract or almond extract

2 teaspoons vanilla sugar-free instant pudding mix

3 packets or ¾ teaspoon stevia (or sweetener of your choice)

¼ - ½ cup water (depending on desired thickness)

5-10 ice cubes (more or less depending on desired thickness)

Place all ingredients in a blender. Mix until desired consistency is reached, scraping sides if necessary.

Yield: 1 serving
Nutritional Analysis: 1 serving equals 273 calories, 5 g fat, 14 g carbohydrate, 43 g protein
Diabetic Exchanges: 2 protein, 1 fat, 1 cheese

Chocolate Covered Cherry

½ cup water

¼ cup 2% cottage cheese

1 scoop Diet Doc Belgian Chocolate protein powder

⅓ cup frozen black cherries

¼ teaspoon cherry extract

¼ teaspoon or 1 packet stevia

2 teaspoons sugar-free instant chocolate pudding mix

5-10 ice cubes (more or less depending on desired thickness)

Place all ingredients in a blender. Mix until desired consistency is reached, scraping sides if necessary.

Yield: 1 serving
Nutritional Analysis: 1 serving equals 234 calories, 4 g fat, 16 g carbohydrate, 33.5 g protein
Diabetic Exchanges: 2 protein, 1 fat, ½ fruit, ½ cheese

Cool Berry

½ cup fat-free plain Greek yogurt

2 tablespoons water

1 scoop Diet Doc Vanilla Bean protein powder

½ cup frozen strawberries

¼ cup fresh or frozen blueberries

5-10 ice cubes (more or less depending on desired thickness)

Place all ingredients in a blender. Mix until desired consistency is reached, scraping sides if necessary.

Yield: 1 serving
Nutritional Analysis: 1 serving equals 271 calories, 3 g fat, 21 g carbohydrate, 40 g protein
Diabetic Exchanges: 1 fruit, 2 protein, 1 fat, ½ milk

Creamy Chocolate Malt

½ cup fat-free cottage cheese

¼ cup water

1 scoop Diet Doc Belgian Chocolate protein powder

2 teaspoons sugar-free instant chocolate pudding mix

5-10 ice cubes (more or less depending on desired thickness)

Place all ingredients in a blender. Mix until desired consistency is reached, scraping sides if necessary.

Yield: 1 serving
Nutritional Analysis: 1 serving equals 263 calories, 3 g fat, 17 g carbohydrate, 42 g protein
Diabetic Exchanges: 2 protein, 1 fat, 1 cheese

Frappuccino Whip

2 cups ice

1.5 cups unsweetened almond milk

2 scoops Diet Doc Vanilla Bean or Belgian Chocolate protein powder

1 cup double-strength coffee (preferably chilled)

1 packet or ¼ teaspoon stevia (or sweetener of choice)

Optional: 2 tablespoons instant coffee granules

Place all ingredients in a blender. Mix until desired consistency is reached, scraping sides if necessary.

Yield: 2 servings
Nutritional Analysis: 1 serving equals 155 calories, 3 g fat, 3 g carbohydrate, 29 g protein
Diabetic Exchanges: 1 protein, 1 milk, ½ fat

Mint Chocolate Madness

½ cup water

½ cup 2% cottage cheese

1 scoop Diet Doc Belgian Chocolate protein blend

½ teaspoon or 2 packets stevia (or sweetener of choice)

1/8 teaspoon mint extract

2 teaspoons sugar-free instant chocolate pudding mix

5-10 ice cubes (more or less depending on desired thickness)

Place all ingredients in a blender. Mix until desired consistency is reached, scraping sides if necessary.

Yield: 1 serving
Nutritional Analysis: 1 serving equals 253.5 calories, 5.5 g fat, 12 g carbohydrate, 39 g protein
Diabetic Exchanges: 2 protein, 1 cheese, 1 fat

Peanut Butter Cup

½ cup water

½ cup 2% cottage cheese

1 scoop Diet Doc Belgian Chocolate protein powder

½ teaspoon or 2 packets stevia (or sweetener of choice)

2 teaspoons natural peanut butter

2 teaspoons sugar-free instant chocolate pudding mix

7-10 ice cubes (more or less depending on desired thickness)

Place all ingredients in a blender. Mix until desired consistency is reached, scraping sides if necessary.

Yield: 1 serving

Nutritional Analysis: 1 serving equals 284 calories, 8 g fat, 13 g carbohydrate, 40 g protein

Diabetic Exchanges: 2 protein, 1 cheese, 1.5 fat

Strawberry Pie

½ cup water

1 scoop Diet Doc Vanilla Bean protein powder

½ cup frozen strawberries

1 whole graham cracker

½ teaspoon or 2 packets stevia (or sweetener of your choice)

5-10 ice cubes (more or less depending on desired thickness)

Place all ingredients in a blender. Mix until desired consistency is reached, scraping sides if necessary.

Yield: 1 serving

Nutritional Analysis: 1 serving equals 246.5 calories, 4.5 g fat, 22 g carbohydrate, 29.5 g protein

Diabetic Exchanges: 2 protein, 1 fat, ½ fruit

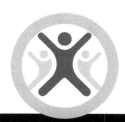

SECTION 6:

Metabolic Inferno Fat-Incinerating Training System

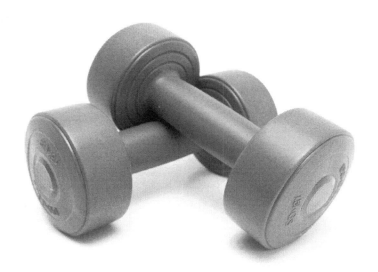

I started lifting weights when I was twelve years old and haven't stopped since. In that time, though, I've wandered through phases of baseball, basketball, softball, martial arts, running, and various fitness fads. Kori's background is similar. Having started in gymnastics, she migrated in and out of various team and individual sports. Once you've had a taste of what being an athlete feels like—the strength, endurance, functionality, and energy—it's hard to stop. And that's a good thing! We call the transition to maintenance *becoming a life athlete* because we hope you too will see that the pursuit of feeling your best is an asset to your health—a lifelong quest. As Kori points out, consistent exercise is also one of the greatest indicators of long-term success.

Creating a training system requires a great deal of thought before the first keystroke can imprint a clean sheet of paper. Hundreds of hours of refinement occur before the first drop of sweat ever hits the pavement. There are far too many great and productive ways of training to claim that we have developed the *only* way, but we wanted to fashion something that would meet the most goals possible—something that we enjoy

doing. Our collective experience and education could have pulled us in many directions, but we came back to a version of how we currently train. Any information flow you ever find yourself in will be influenced by the context of the time period and you'll see this is no different. There are good reasons that functional and athletic movements have infiltrated the fitness industry and you'll see a great deal of them mixed into this system. We also include a necessary foundation: traditional strength training and cardiovascular conditioning to enhance maximal results.

Other variables that we considered are ease of use, appropriate progressions, and including varying fitness levels.

Health and participation requirements

We recommend you see your physician for an okay to participate in this program. Plenty of instructions and warnings are included throughout, but I'll repeat a formal one here: You are accepting full responsibility for ensuring that you are healthy enough to participate in an exercise program and have taken it upon yourself to notify and ask your physician for permission. Not to scare you; we really have taken significant steps to make sure this is safe and progresses slowly, per your ability, but we don't know your health and medical history. Your doctor may have specific instructions for you.

Equipment needs

Much of the training can be done with no equipment at all—just you, a towel, and a bottle of water. Progressions do include use of exercise bands/tubing, weighted medicine balls, a stability ball, and dumbbells. All of these items can be found in the sporting goods department at Wal-Mart, Target, or any sporting goods store with very little investment. The value they bring to your ability to move into higher levels of function are great enough for us to include them. The hardcore gym enthusiast will find that these exercises can be done in a gym with equipment as well. We often create programs with these same components for high-level athletes to perform in training facilities.

Protocol description

Day 1: Upper-body – functional workout

Day 2: Lower-body – strength workout

Day 3: Steady-state cardio and ab workout

Day 4: Upper-body – strength workout

Day 5: Lower-body – functional workout

Day 6: High-intensity cardio and ab workout

Day 7: Recovery – active rest

There are two pure strength days: an upper- and lower-body split. Those are days that the quality of muscle contraction and good form should be utilized to condition your muscle and keep joints injury free. We want you to progress in strength, but you need reps, sets, workouts, and weeks of conditioning to prepare your body for more aggressive work. Don't worry, you will see results early and your muscle will begin taking shape.

The two functional workouts also focus on upper- and lower-body separately, but high-level athletic movements are mixed in to add conditioning and accelerated athletic progress. Be careful to move through the progressions slowly, from beginner to intermediate and to advanced; each week evolves in difficulty. This gives you two ways to advance.

Cardiovascular conditioning is broken into steady-state and interval training and abdominal work is mixed in both days. Seeing those abs takes more than doing crunches—losing the body fat through a combination of overall fat loss be way of diet and exercise is necessary—but we include plenty of core work because it's important for safety and overall physical health. One thing to note about the cardiovascular workouts is that the interval training can get aggressive. Be sure you're monitoring your heart rate either with a heart-rate monitor (also found in sporting goods stores) or the 'ole standby method of checking your pulse with your finger, counting for 6 seconds, and multiplying by 10. Maximum heart rate is 220 minus your age and we use a percent of that to allow you to gauge your effort level. Never, ever feel you are tied to those numbers if you feel it's too much, too soon. Back off and go at your own pace.

Phases of progress

Weeks 1 and 2:

The focus during the first two weeks is to slowly build exercise tolerance and intensity. Creating a safe and productive foundation of strength and performance will lead to weeks of progress—and hopefully years if we can talk you into sticking with it! Combined with the nutrition plan, the frequency and completeness of training will promote glycogen depletion, which will accelerate body fat loss.

Weeks 3 and 4:

Weeks three and four will be progressive in functionality, effort, and intensity. Weight training movements are incorporated with cardiovascular work in creative, purposeful ways. Strength and energy will increase as body fat losses continue. Advanced movements are introduced in week four and more complex function movements begin to enhance athleticism.

Week 5:

Cardivascular work progresses during week five to keep fat mobilization moving forward at the same time training advances.

Week 6:

More variety is introduced in week six to expand exercise knowledge and experience while core strength is emphasized. Progress continues toward becoming an athlete for life!

Week 7:

The final week integrates program designs previously performed with movement advancements as a set up for future programming. The length of training sessions has been building throughout the program and weeks six and seven are designed to challenge!

Day 50:

Plan for permanence! The program can be repeated by moving through the progression levels. You can also visit our website for advanced programming options—progress doesn't have to stop; you're just getting started!

Week 1 Day 1: Upper Body Functional Training

10-minute light cardiovascular warm up such as walking or stationary bike.

SUPERSET 1

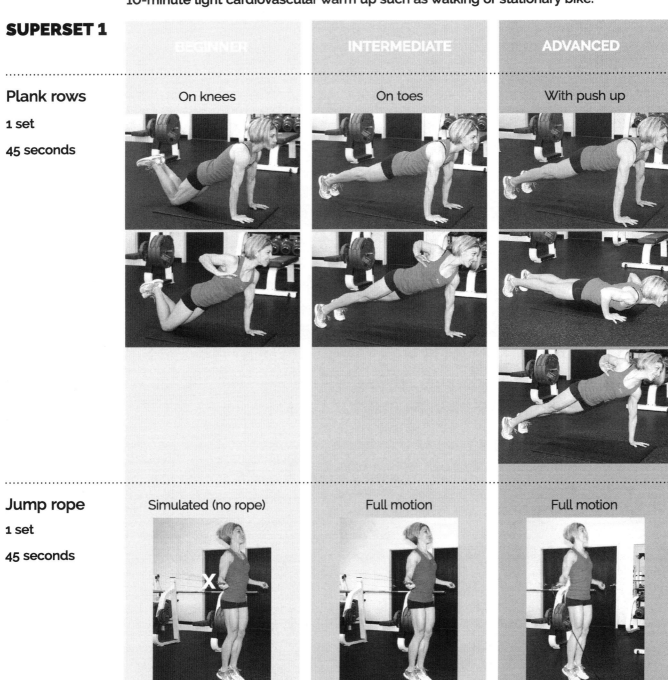

	BEGINNER	INTERMEDIATE	ADVANCED
Plank rows 1 set 45 seconds	On knees	On toes	With push up
Jump rope 1 set 45 seconds	Simulated (no rope)	Full motion	Full motion

REST 30 seconds

SUPERSET 2

	BEGINNER	INTERMEDIATE	ADVANCED

Pushups

1 set

45 seconds

Against wall	On knees	On toes

High knees

1 set

30 seconds

Walk through	Knees to waist	Knees to chest

REST 30 seconds

SUPERSET 3

	BEGINNER	INTERMEDIATE	ADVANCED
Bicep band curls 1 set 45 seconds	Light resistance 	Medium resistance 	Heavy resistance
Jump rope 1 set 30 seconds	Simulated (no rope) 	Full motion 	Full motion

REST 30 seconds

SUPERSET 4

		INTERMEDIATE	ADVANCED

Tricep band kickbacks

1 set

45 seconds

Light resistance	Medium resistance	Heavy resistance
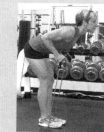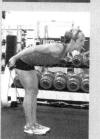	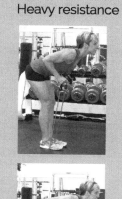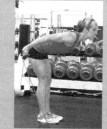	

Mountain climbers

1 set

30 seconds

Standing	Walk through	Full motion
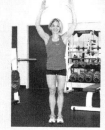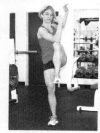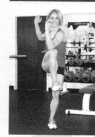	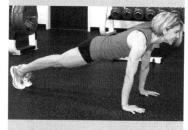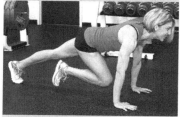	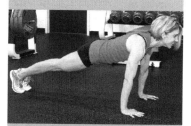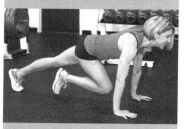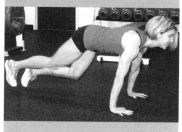

REST 30 seconds

repeat cycle 2x	repeat cycle 3x	repeat cycle 4x

Week **1** Day **2**: Lower body Strength Circuit

10-minute light cardiovascular warm up such as walking or stationary bike.

CIRCUIT

	BEGINNER	INTERMEDIATE	ADVANCED
Squats 1 set 20 reps	Half squat	Full squat	DB squat
Stiff-legged dead lifts 1 set 20 reps	No weight	Light DBs	Medium DBs

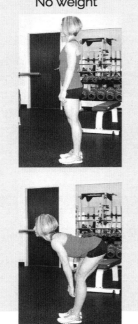

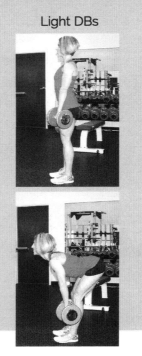

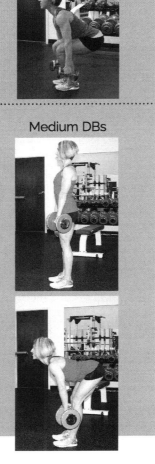

		INTERMEDIATE	ADVANCED
Goblet squats 1 set 20 reps	Half squat 	Full squat 	DB squat
Stability ball hamstring curl 1 set 20 reps	Curl only 	Curl and contract 	Curl and bridge

REST 60 seconds

repeat cycle 2x   repeat cycle 3x   repeat cycle 4x

INCREASE WEIGHT PER ROUND AS TOLERATED

Week 1 Day 3: Steady-State Cardio & Abs

10-minute light cardiovascular warm up such as walking or stationary bike.

• Stretch slowly for 10 minutes: hamstrings, quads, glutes/hips, calves.

• 30 minutes of cardiovascular work at 60 percent of maximum heart rate (220 minus your age is your maximum heart rate).

• You may vary cardio type or stay with one form of exercise for the 30-minute session.

• Monitor heart rate closely as suggestions for intensity increase. At no time are you required to work at a level that you feel is unsafe. Decrease intensity or duration as necessary and progress at your own pace. We would suggest trying to focus on duration even if intensity needs to be dropped to an easier level. It would be better to walk slowly for 30 minutes than start out too fast and have to stop.

SUPERSET 1

	BEGINNER	INTERMEDIATE	ADVANCED
Crunches 1 set 30 seconds	Knees bent	Pause	Add reach
Reverse crunches 1 set 30 seconds	Knees to chest	Lift hips	Pause

REST 30 seconds

SUPERSET 2

		INTERMEDIATE	ADVANCED

Medicine ball toe touches

1 set

30 seconds

Knees bent

Arms extended

Heavier ball

V-ups

1 set

30 seconds

Hands on floor

Balancing/partial

Full motion

REST 30 seconds

SUPERSET 3

	BEGINNER	INTERMEDIATE	ADVANCED
Seated med ball Russian twists 1 set 30 seconds	Hands close to body	Arms extended	Heavier ball (or feet elevated)
Bicycle crunches 1 set 30 seconds	Slow, knees bent	Extend leg	Pause

REST 30 sec

repeat cycle 2x   repeat cycle 3x   repeat cycle 4x

Week 1 Day 4: Upper Body Strength Circuit

10-minute light cardiovascular warm up such as walking or stationary bike.

CIRCUIT

		INTERMEDIATE	ADVANCED

1-arm row

1 set

20 reps

Light DB | Medium DB | Heavy DB

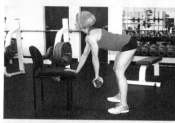 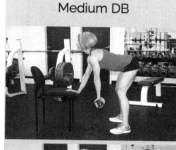 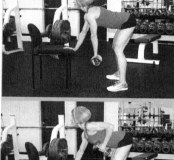

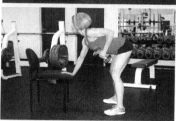 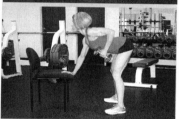 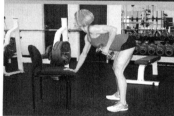

Stability ball chest press

1 set

20 reps

Light DB | Medium DB | Heavy DB

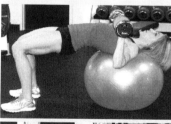 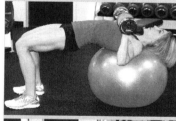 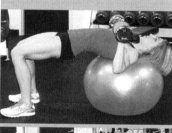

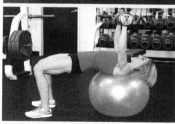 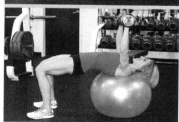 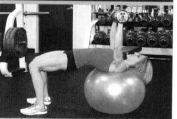

	BEGINNER	INTERMEDIATE	ADVANCED
Shoulder lateral 1 set 20 reps	No weight	Light DB	Medium DB
Overhead tricep extension 1 set 20 reps	Light DB	Medium DB	Medium DB

Bicep curl

1 set

20 reps

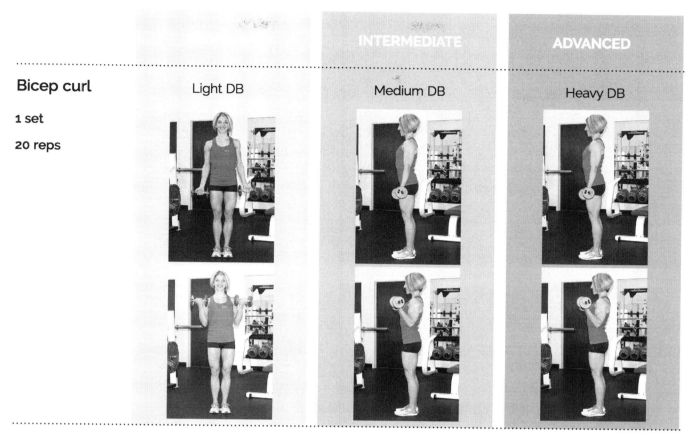

| Light DB | INTERMEDIATE
Medium DB | ADVANCED
Heavy DB |

REST 30 seconds

repeat cycle 2x   repeat cycle 3x   repeat cycle 4x

INCREASE WEIGHT PER ROUND AS TOLERATED

Week 1 Day 5: Lower Body Functional Training

10-minute light cardiovascular warm up such as walking or stationary bike.

SUPERSET 1

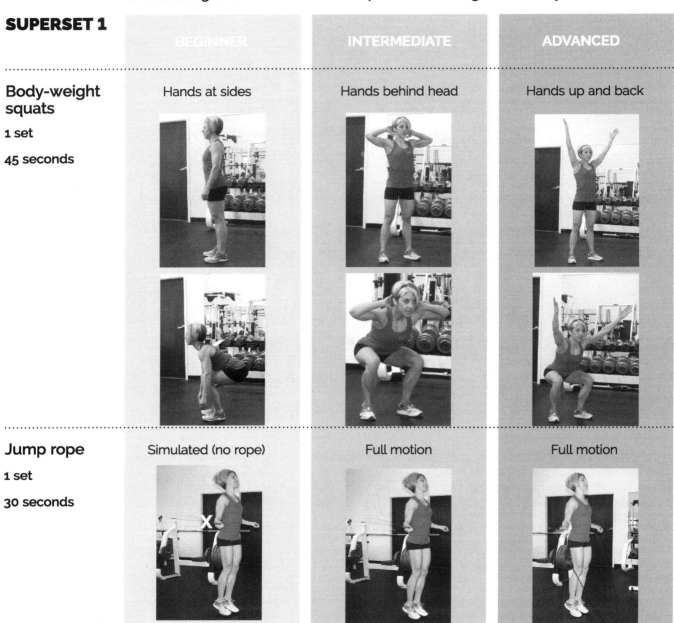

	BEGINNER	INTERMEDIATE	ADVANCED
Body-weight squats 1 set 45 seconds	Hands at sides	Hands behind head	Hands up and back
Jump rope 1 set 30 seconds	Simulated (no rope)	Full motion	Full motion

REST 30 seconds

SUPERSET 2

		INTERMEDIATE	ADVANCED

Side lunges

1 set

45 seconds

Step out	Half lunge	Full lunge

Pushup plank spidermans

1 set

45 seconds

Standing	On knees	Full motion

REST 30 seconds

SUPERSET 3

	BEGINNER	INTERMEDIATE	ADVANCED
Sumo squat 1 set 45 seconds	Partial squat 	Half squat 	Full squat
Jump rope 1 set 30 seconds	Simulated (no rope) 	Full motion 	Full motion

REST 30 seconds

SUPERSET 4

	BEGINNER	INTERMEDIATE	ADVANCED

Alternating lunges

1 set

45 seconds

Partial lunge	Half lunge	Full lunge

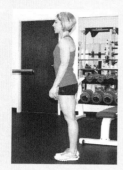 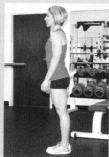 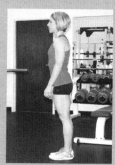

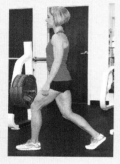 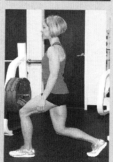 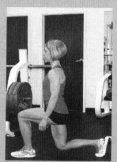

Pushup plank lateral hops

1 set

30 seconds

Plank only	Step out	Full motion

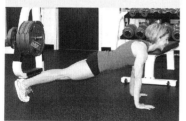 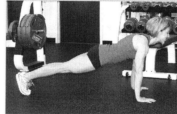 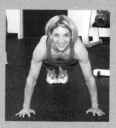

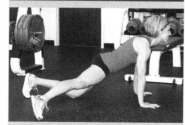 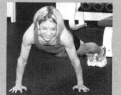

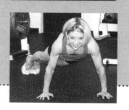

REST 30 seconds

repeat cycle 2x   repeat cycle 3x   repeat cycle 4x

Week **1** Day**6**: High-Intensity Interval Cardio & Abs

10-minute light cardiovascular warm up such as walking or stationary bike.

- Stretch slowly for 10 minutes: hamstrings, quads, glutes/hips, calves.
- You may use any cardio form such as jogging, elliptical, or bike.

CIRCUIT	BEGINNER	INTERMEDIATE	ADVANCED
Cardio interval 60 seconds	Bike	Elliptical	Jog or functional movement
Active rest 60 seconds			
Cardio interval 45 seconds	Bike	Elliptical	Jog or functional movement
Active rest 45 seconds			
Cardio interval 30 seconds	Bike	Elliptical	Jog or functional movement
Active rest 30 seconds			
Cardio interval 15 seconds	Bike	Elliptical	Jog or functional movement
Active rest 15 seconds			

REST 60 seconds

SUPERSET 1

| | | INTERMEDIATE | ADVANCED |

Crunches

1 set

60 seconds

Reverse crunches

1 set

60 seconds

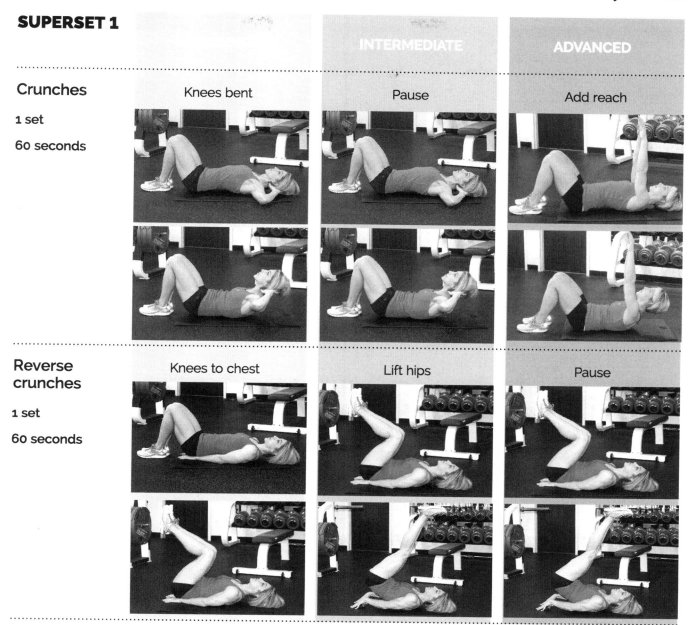

| | Knees bent | Pause | Add reach |
| Crunches | | | |

| | Knees to chest | Lift hips | Pause |
| Reverse crunches | | | |

REST 60 seconds

SUPERSET 2

	BEGINNER	INTERMEDIATE	ADVANCED

Mountain climbers

1 set

45 seconds

Plank

1 set

45 seconds

On knees	On toes	One-armed

REST 45 seconds

SUPERSET 3

		INTERMEDIATE	ADVANCED
Stability ball knee-ins 1 set 30 seconds	Half rep 	Knees to chest 	Pikes
Stability ball Russian twists 1 set 30 seconds	Use hands to balance 	Arms extended 	Hold med ball

REST 30 seconds

repeat cycle 1x   repeat cycle 2x   repeat cycle 3x

Week **2** Day **1**: Upper Body Functional Training

10-minute light cardiovascular warm up such as walking or stationary bike.

SUPERSET 1

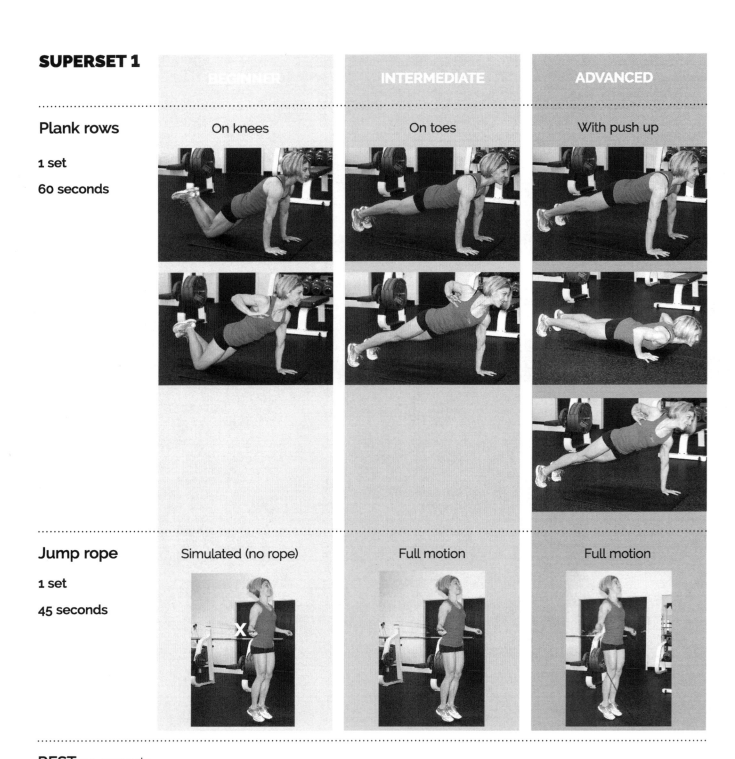

	BEGINNER	INTERMEDIATE	ADVANCED
Plank rows 1 set 60 seconds	On knees	On toes	With push up
Jump rope 1 set 45 seconds	Simulated (no rope)	Full motion	Full motion

REST 30 seconds

SUPERSET 2

		INTERMEDIATE	ADVANCED
Pushups 1 set 60 seconds	Against wall	On knees	On toes
High knees 1 set 45 seconds	Walk through	Knees to waist	Knees to chest

REST 30 seconds

SUPERSET 3

	BEGINNER	INTERMEDIATE	ADVANCED
Bicep band curls 1 set 60 seconds	Light resistance	Medium resistance	Heavy resistance
Jump rope 1 set 45 seconds	Simulated (no rope)	Full motion	Full motion

REST 30 seconds

SUPERSET 4

		INTERMEDIATE	ADVANCED

Tricep band kickbacks

1 set

45 seconds

Light resistance	Medium resistance	Heavy resistance
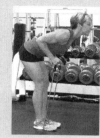	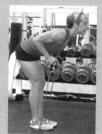	
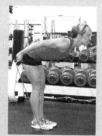	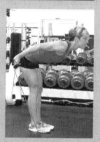	

Mountain climbers

1 set

30 seconds

Standing	Walk through	Full motion
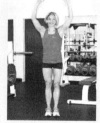	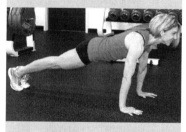	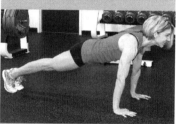
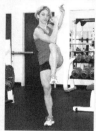	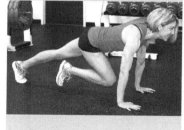	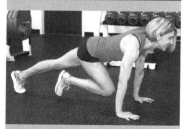
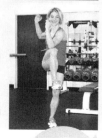		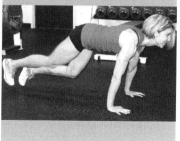

REST 30 seconds	repeat cycle 1x	repeat cycle 2x	repeat cycle 3x

Week 2 Day 2: Lower body Strength Circuit

10-minute light cardiovascular warm up such as walking or stationary bike.

CIRCUIT

	BEGINNER	INTERMEDIATE	ADVANCED
Squats 1 set 15 reps	Half squat 	Full squat 	DB squat
Stiff-legged dead lifts 1 set 15 reps	No weight 	Light DBs 	Medium DBs

		INTERMEDIATE	ADVANCED
Goblet squats 1 set 15 reps	Half squat	Full squat	DB squat
Stability ball hamstring curl 1 set 15 reps	Curl only	Curl and contract	Curl and bridge

REST 60 seconds

repeat cycle 3x   repeat cycle 4x   repeat cycle 5x

INCREASE WEIGHT PER ROUND AS TOLERATED

Week 2 Day 3: Steady-State Cardio & Abs

10-minute light cardiovascular warm up such as walking or stationary bike.

• Stretch slowly for 10 minutes: hamstrings, quads, glutes/hips, calves.

• 30 minutes of cardiovascular work at 65 percent of maximum heart rate (220 minus your age is your maximum heart rate).

• You may vary cardio type or stay with one form of exercise for the 30-minute session.

• Monitor heart rate closely as suggestions for intensity increase. At no time are you required to work at a level that you feel is unsafe. Decrease intensity or duration as necessary and progress at your own pace. We would suggest trying to focus on duration even if intensity needs to be dropped to an easier level. It would be better to walk slowly for 30 minutes than start out too fast and have to stop.

SUPERSET 1

	BEGINNER	INTERMEDIATE	ADVANCED
Crunches 1 set 45 seconds	Knees bent	Pause	Add reach
Reverse crunches 1 set 30 seconds	Knees to chest	Lift hips	Pause

REST 30 seconds

SUPERSET 2

	BEGINNER	INTERMEDIATE	ADVANCED

Medicine ball toe touches

1 set

45 seconds

Knees bent	Arms extended	Heavier ball

V-ups

1 set

30 seconds

Hands on floor	Balance/partial motion	Full motion

REST 30 seconds

SUPERSET 3

	BEGINNER	INTERMEDIATE	ADVANCED

Seated med ball Russian twists

1 set

45 seconds

Hands close to body	Arms extended	Heavier ball

Bicycle crunches

1 set

30 seconds

Slow, knees bent	Extend legs	Pause

REST 30 seconds

repeat cycle 2x	repeat cycle 3x	repeat cycle 4x

Week **2** Day**4**: Upper Body Strength Circuit

10-minute light cardiovascular warm up such as walking or stationary bike.

CIRCUIT

		INTERMEDIATE	ADVANCED

1-arm row

1 set

15 reps

Light DB	Medium DB	Heavy DB

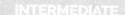
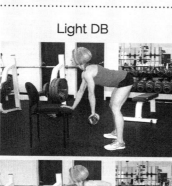
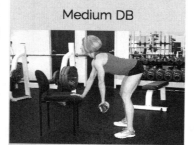
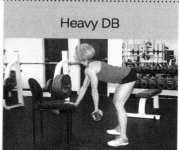
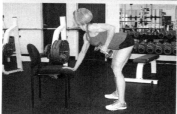
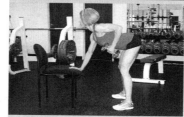
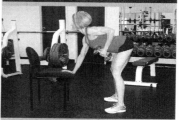

Stability ball chest press

1 set

15 reps

Light DB	Medium DB	Heavy DB

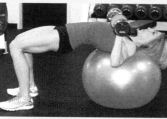
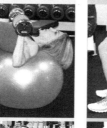
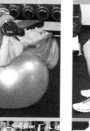
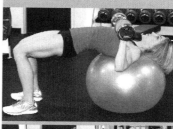
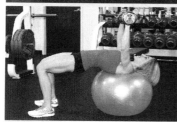
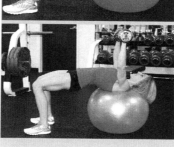
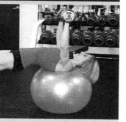
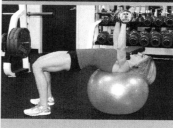

	BEGINNER	INTERMEDIATE	ADVANCED
Shoulder lateral **1 set** **15 reps**	Light DB	Medium DB	Heavy DB
Overhead tricep extension **1 set** **15 reps**	Light DB	Medium DB	Heavy DB

INTERMEDIATE

ADVANCED

Bicep curl

1 set

15 reps

Light DB

Medium DB

Heavy DB

REST 45 seconds

repeat cycle 3x

repeat cycle 4x

repeat cycle 5x

INCREASE WEIGHT PER ROUND AS TOLERATED

Week 2 Day 5: Lower Body Functional Training

10-minute light cardiovascular warm up such as walking or stationary bike.

SUPERSET 1

	BEGINNER	INTERMEDIATE	ADVANCED
Body-weight squats 1 set 60 Seconds	Hands at sides	Hands behind head	Hands up and back
Jump rope 1 set 45 seconds	Simulated (no rope)	Full motion	Full motion

REST 30 seconds

SUPERSET 2

	INTERMEDIATE	ADVANCED

Side lunges

1 set

60 seconds

Step out | Half lunge | Full lunge

Pushup plank spidermans

1 set

45 seconds

Standing | On knees | Full motion

REST 30 seconds

SUPERSET 3

	BEGINNER	INTERMEDIATE	ADVANCED
Sumo squat 1 set 60 seconds	Partial squat 	Half squat 	Full squat
Jump rope 1 set 45 seconds	Simulated (no rope) 	Full motion 	Full motion

REST 30 seconds

SUPERSET 4

		INTERMEDIATE	ADVANCED

Alternating lunges

1 set

60 seconds

Partial lunge

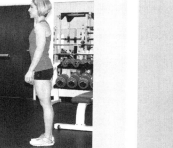
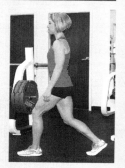

Half lunge

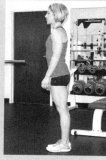
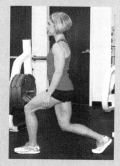

Full lunge

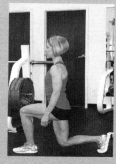

Pushup plank lateral hops

1 set

45 seconds

Plank only

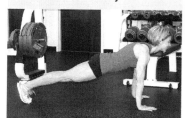

Step out

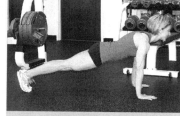
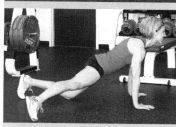

Full motion

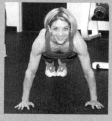
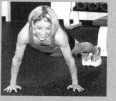
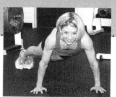

REST 30 seconds

repeat cycle 3x   repeat cycle 4x   repeat cycle 5x

Week 2 Day 6: High-Intensity Interval Cardio & Abs

10-minute light cardiovascular warm up such as walking or stationary bike.

• Stretch slowly for 10 minutes: hamstrings, quads, glutes/hips, calves.

• You may use any cardio form such as jogging, elliptical, or bike.

CIRCUIT	BEGINNER	INTERMEDIATE	ADVANCED
Cardio interval 1 x 60 sec.	Bike	Elliptical	Jog or functional movement
Active rest 1 x 60 sec.			
Cardio interval 2 x 45 sec.	Bike	Elliptical	Jog or functional movement
Active rest 2 x 45 sec.			
Cardio interval 3 x 30 sec.	Bike	Elliptical	Jog or functional movement
Active rest 3 x 30 sec.			
Cardio interval 4 x 15 sec.	Bike	Elliptical	Jog or functional movement
Active rest 4 x 15 sec.			

REST 60 seconds

TRI-SET 1

		INTERMEDIATE	**ADVANCED**
Crunches 1 set 60 seconds	Knees bent	Pause	Add reach
Reverse crunches 1 set 60 seconds	Knees to chest	Lift hips	Pause

	BEGINNER	INTERMEDIATE	ADVANCED
Mountain climbers 1 set 30 seconds	Standing 	Walk through 	Full motion

REST 60 seconds

TRI-SET 2

	BEGINNER	INTERMEDIATE	ADVANCED
Spidermans 1 set 45 seconds	Plank 	Knees out 	Add hop
Plank 1 set 45 seconds	On knees 	On toes 	One-armed

		INTERMEDIATE	ADVANCED
Mountain climbers 1 set 30 seconds	Standing	Walk through	Full motion
Stability ball knee-ins 1 set 30 seconds	Half rep	Knees to chest	Pikes

REST 45 seconds

TRI-SET 3

	BEGINNER	INTERMEDIATE	ADVANCED

Stability ball Russian twists

1 set

30 seconds

Use hands to balance
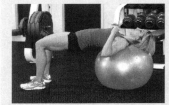
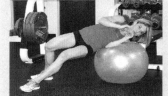
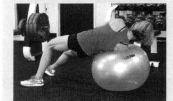

Arms extended
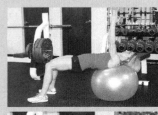
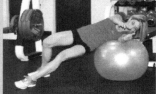
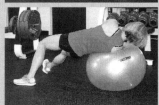

Hold med ball
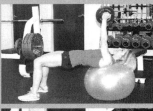
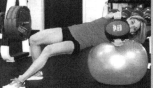
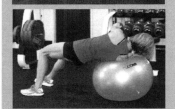

Mountain climbers

1 set

30 seconds

Standing
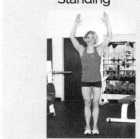
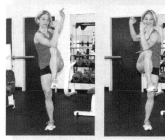

Walk through
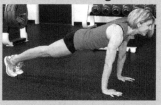
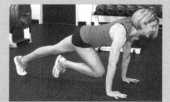

Full motion
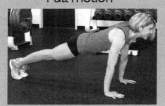
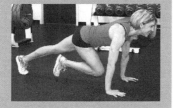
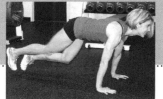

REST 30 seconds

Week 3 Day 1: Upper Body Functional Training

10-minute light cardiovascular warm up such as walking or stationary bike.

GIANT SET 1

		INTERMEDIATE	ADVANCED
Jump rope 1 set 60 seconds	Simulated (no rope)	Full motion	Full motion
Plank rows 1 set 45 seconds	On knees	On toes	With pushup

	BEGINNER	INTERMEDIATE	ADVANCED
Bicep band curls 1 set 45 seconds	Light resistance	Medium resistance	Heavy resistance
Pushup position lateral hops 1 set 30 seconds	On knees/lateral taps	On toes/feet apart	On toes/feet together

REST 30 seconds

GIANT SET 2

		INTERMEDIATE	ADVANCED

Jump rope

1 set

60 seconds

Simulated (no rope)

Full motion

Full motion

Pushups

1 set

45 seconds

Against wall

On knees

On toes

	BEGINNER	INTERMEDIATE	ADVANCED
Tricep band kickbacks **1 set** **45 seconds**	Light resistance 	Medium resistance 	Heavy resistance
Pushup plank front/back hops **1 set** **30 seconds**	On elbows 	Walk through 	Full motion
REST 30 seconds	repeat cycle 2x	repeat cycle 3x	repeat cycle 4x

Week 3 Day 2: Lower Body Strength Circuit

10-minute light cardiovascular warm up such as walking or stationary bike.

CIRCUIT

		INTERMEDIATE	ADVANCED
Squats 1 set 20 reps	Half squat	Full squat	DB squat
Stiff-legged dead lift 1 set 20 reps	No weight	Light DBs	Medium DBs

	BEGINNER	INTERMEDIATE	ADVANCED
Step-ups **1 set** **20 reps**	No weight	Light DBs	Medium DBs

	INTERMEDIATE	ADVANCED

Stability ball hamstring curl

1 set

20 reps

Curl only	Curl and contract	Curl and bridge

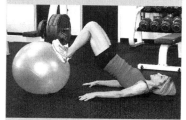
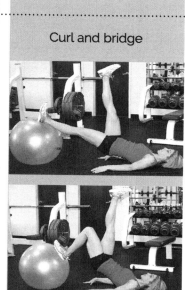

Goblet squats

1 set

20 reps

Half squat	Full squat	DB squat

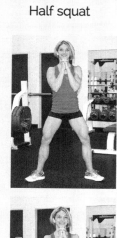
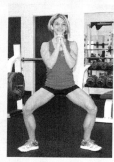
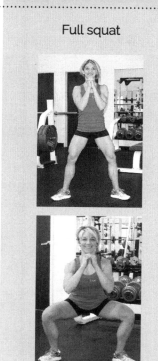
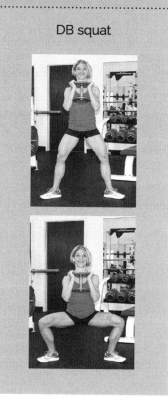

	BEGINNER	INTERMEDIATE	ADVANCED
Band hamstring curl **1 set** **20 reps**	Light resistance	Medium resistance	Heavy resistance

REST 60 seconds   repeat cycle 2x   repeat cycle 3x   repeat cycle 4x

Week 3 Day 3: Steady-State Cardio & Abs

10-minute light cardiovascular warm up such as walking or stationary bike.

- Stretch slowly for 10 minutes: hamstrings, quads, glutes/hips, calves.

- 40 minutes of cardiovascular work at 60 percent of maximum heart rate (220 minus your age is your maximum heart rate).

- You may vary cardio type or stay with one form of exercise for the 40-minute session.

- Monitor heart rate closely as suggestions for intensity increase. At no time are you required to work at a level that you feel is unsafe. Decrease intensity or duration as necessary and progress at your own pace. We would suggest trying to focus on duration even if intensity needs to be dropped to an easier level. It would be better to walk slowly for 40 minutes than start out too fast and have to stop.

TRI-SET 1

		INTERMEDIATE	ADVANCED
V-ups 1 set 30 seconds	Hands on floor	Balance, partial motion	Full motion

	BEGINNER	INTERMEDIATE	ADVANCED
Reverse crunches 1 set 30 seconds	Knees to chest	Lift hips	Pause
Medicine ball toe touches 1 set 30 seconds	Knees bent	Arms extended	Heavier ball

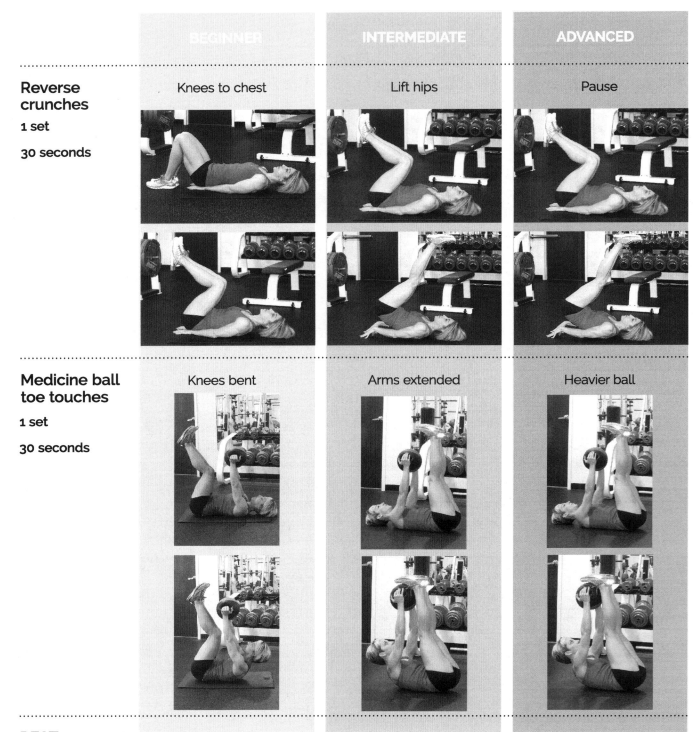

REST 30 seconds

TRI-SET 2

Crunches

1 set

30 seconds

Knees bent	Pause	Add reach

Seated med ball Russian twists

1 set

30 seconds

Hands close to body	Arms extended	Heavier ball or feet elevated

	BEGINNER	INTERMEDIATE	ADVANCED

Bicycle crunches

1 set

30 seconds

Slow, knees bent	Extend legs	Pause

REST 30 seconds

repeat cycle 1x	repeat cycle 2x	repeat cycle 3x

Week 3 Day 4: Upper Body Strength Circuit

10-minute light cardiovascular warm up such as walking or stationary bike.

CIRCUIT

	BEGINNER	INTERMEDIATE	ADVANCED

1-arm row

1 set

30 seconds

Light DB	Medium DB	Heavy DB

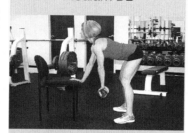 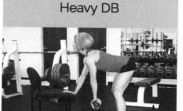
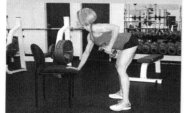 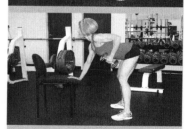

Rear lateral

1 set

30 seconds

Light DB	Medium DB	Heavy DB

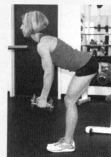 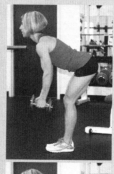 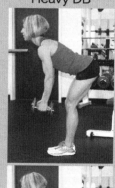
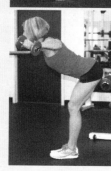 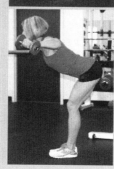 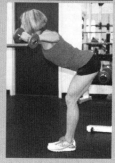

	BEGINNER	INTERMEDIATE	ADVANCED
Stability ball chest press 1 set 20 reps	Light DB	Medium DB	Heavy DB
Stability ball fly 1 set 20 reps	Light DB	Medium DB	Heavy DB

		INTERMEDIATE	ADVANCED

Overhead tricep extension

1 set

20 reps

Light DB	Medium DB	Heavy DB

Bicep curl

1 set

20 reps

Light DB	Medium DB	Heavy DB

REST 45 seconds

repeat cycle 2x	repeat cycle 3x	repeat cycle 4x

INCREASE WEIGHT PER ROUND AS TOLERATED

Week 3 Day 5: Lower Body Functional Training

10-minute light cardiovascular warm up such as walking or stationary bike.

CIRCUIT 1

	BEGINNER	INTERMEDIATE	ADVANCED
Jump rope 1 set 60 seconds	Simulated (no rope) 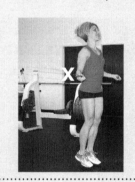	Full motion 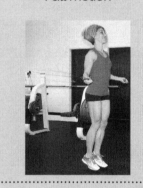	Full motion 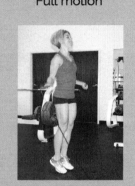
Body-weight squats 1 set 45 seconds	Hands at sides 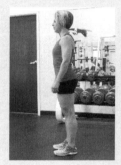 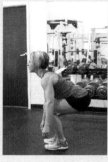	Hands behind head 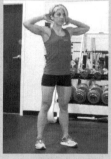 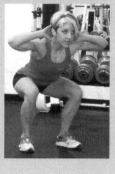	Hands up and back 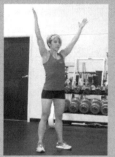 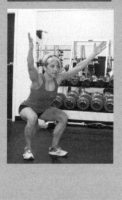

		INTERMEDIATE	**ADVANCED**
Side lunges 1 set 45 seconds	Step out	Half lunge	Full lunge

Pushup plank spidermans 1 set 30 seconds	Standing	On knees	Full motion

REST 30 seconds

CIRCUIT 2

	BEGINNER	INTERMEDIATE	ADVANCED
Jump rope 1 set 60 seconds	Simulated (no rope) 	Full motion 	Full motion
Sumo squat 1 set 45 seconds	Partial squat 	Half squat 	Full squat

	INTERMEDIATE	ADVANCED
Alternating lunges 1 set 45 seconds	Partial lunge	Half lunge	Full lunge

	INTERMEDIATE	ADVANCED
Pushup plank lateral hops 1 set 30 seconds	Plank only	Step out	Full motion

REST 30 seconds

repeat cycle 2x repeat cycle 3x repeat cycle 4x

Week 3 Day 6: High-Intensity Interval Cardio & Abs

10-minute light cardiovascular warm up such as walking or stationary bike.

- Stretch slowly for 10 minutes: hamstrings, quads, glutes/hips, calves.
- You may use any cardio form such as jogging, elliptical, or bike.
- As intervals shorten, intensity should increase.
- Active rest example: walk.

CIRCUIT	BEGINNER	INTERMEDIATE	ADVANCED
Cardio interval 2 x 60 sec.	Bike	Elliptical	Jog or functional movement
Active rest 2 x 30 sec.			
Cardio interval 3 x 50 sec.	Bike	Elliptical	Jog or functional movement
Active rest 3 x 25 sec.			
Cardio interval 4 x 40 sec.	Bike	Elliptical	Jog or functional movement
Active rest 4 x 20 sec.			
Cardio interval 5 x 30 sec.	Bike	Elliptical	Jog or functional movement
Active rest 5 x 15 sec.			

REST 60 seconds

TRI-SET 1

		INTERMEDIATE	ADVANCED
Crunches 1 set 60 seconds	Knees bent	Pause	Add reach
Reverse crunches 1 set 60 seconds	Knees to chest	Lift hips	Pause

	BEGINNER	INTERMEDIATE	ADVANCED

Cross-body mountain climbers

1 set

30 seconds

	Standing	Walk through	Full motion

REST 30 seconds

TRI-SET 2

		INTERMEDIATE	ADVANCED
Spidermans 1 set 60 seconds	Plank 	Knees out 	Add hop
Plank 1 set 60 seconds	On knees 	On toes 	One-armed

Cross-body mountain climbers

1 set

30 seconds

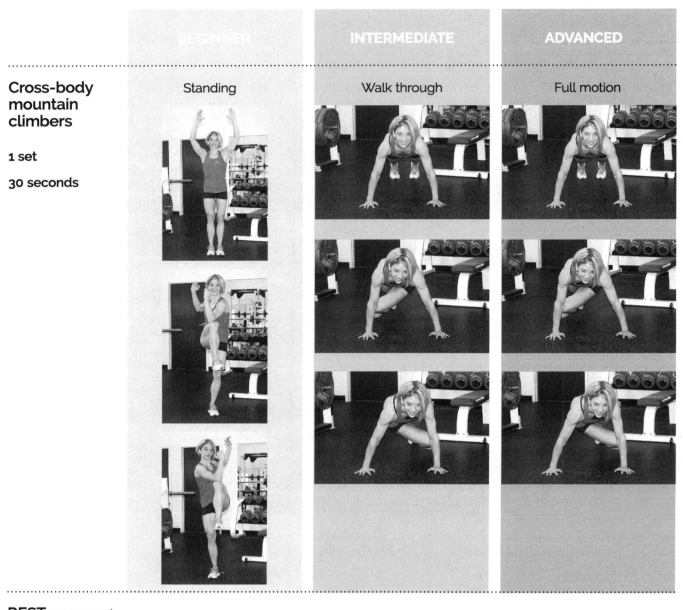

BEGINNER	INTERMEDIATE	ADVANCED
Standing	Walk through	Full motion

REST 30 seconds

TRI-SET 3

	BEGINNER	INTERMEDIATE	ADVANCED
Stability ball knee-ins 1 set 60 seconds	Half rep	Knees to chest	Pike
Med ball Russian twists 1 set 60 seconds	Hands close to body	Arms extended	Heavier ball or feet elevated

	BEGINNER	INTERMEDIATE	ADVANCED
Cross-body mountain climbers **1 set** **30 seconds**	Standing	Walk through	Full motion

REST 30 seconds

repeat cycle 1x   repeat cycle 2x   repeat cycle 3x

Week 4 Day 1: Upper Body Functional Training

10-minute light cardiovascular warm up such as walking or stationary bike.

GIANT SET 1

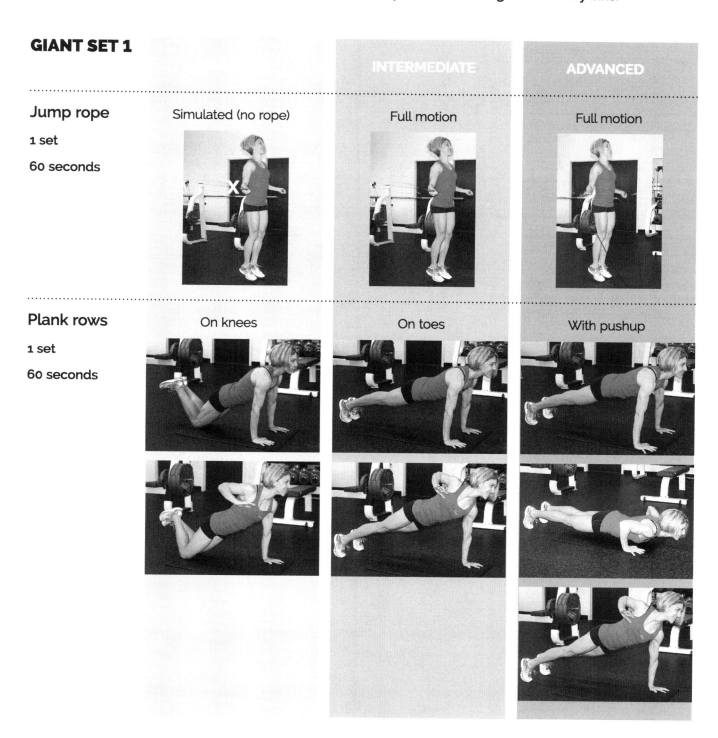

		INTERMEDIATE	ADVANCED
Jump rope 1 set 60 seconds	Simulated (no rope)	Full motion	Full motion
Plank rows 1 set 60 seconds	On knees	On toes	With pushup

	BEGINNER	INTERMEDIATE	ADVANCED
Bicep band curls **1 set** **60 seconds**	Light resistance	Medium resistance	Heavy resistance
Pushup plank lateral hops **1 set** **45 seconds**	On knees/lateral taps	On toes/feet apart	On toes/feet together

REST 30 seconds

GIANT SET 2

		INTERMEDIATE	ADVANCED
Jump rope 1 set 60 seconds	Simulated (no rope)	Full motion	Full motion
Pushups 1 set 60 seconds	Against wall	On knees	On toes

	BEGINNER	INTERMEDIATE	ADVANCED

Tricep band kickbacks

1 set

60 seconds

	Light resistance	Medium resistance	Heavy resistance

Pushup plank front/back hops

1 set

45 seconds

	On elbows	Walk through	Full motion

REST 30 seconds

repeat cycle 3x   repeat cycle 4x   repeat cycle 5x

Week 4 Day 2: Lower Body Strength Circuit

10-minute light cardiovascular warm up such as walking or stationary bike.

CIRCUIT		INTERMEDIATE	ADVANCED
Squats 1 set 15 reps	Half squat 	Full squat 	DB squat
Stiff-legged dead lift 1 set 15 reps	No weight 	Light DBs 	Medium DBs

Step-ups

1 set

15 reps

BEGINNER	INTERMEDIATE	ADVANCED
No weight	Light DBs	Medium DBs

	INTERMEDIATE	ADVANCED
Stability ball hamstring curl **1 set** **15 reps**	Curl only	Curl and contract	Curl and bridge

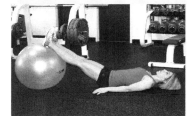
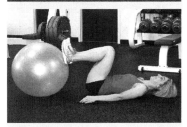
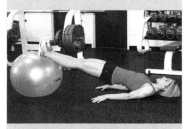
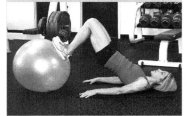
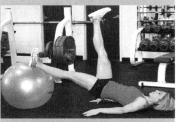
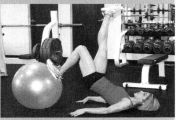

Goblet squats **1 set** **15 reps**	Half squat	Full squat	DB squat

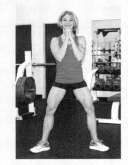
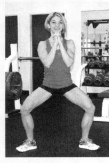
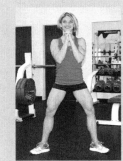
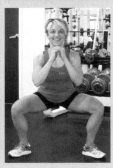
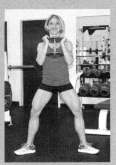
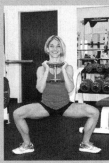

Band hamstring curl

1 set

15 reps

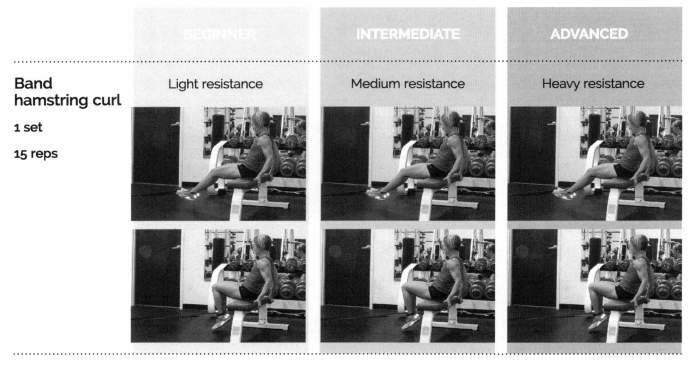

BEGINNER	INTERMEDIATE	ADVANCED
Light resistance	Medium resistance	Heavy resistance

REST 60 seconds

repeat cycle 3x   repeat cycle 4x   repeat cycle 5x

INCREASE WEIGHT PER ROUND AS TOLERATED

Week **4** Day **3**: Steady-State Cardio & Abs

10-minute light cardiovascular warm up such as walking or stationary bike.

• Stretch slowly for 10 minutes: hamstrings, quads, glutes/hips, calves.

• 40 minutes of cardiovascular work at 65 percent of maximum heart rate (220 minus your age is your maximum heart rate).

• You may vary cardio type or stay with one form of exercise for the 40-minute session.

• Monitor heart rate closely as suggestions for intensity increase. At no time are you required to work at a level that you feel is unsafe. Decrease intensity or duration as necessary and progress at your own pace. We would suggest trying to focus on duration even if intensity needs to be dropped to an easier level. It would be better to walk slowly for 40 minutes than start out too fast and have to stop.

TRI-SET 1

	BEGINNER	INTERMEDIATE	ADVANCED
V-ups 1 set 45 seconds	Hands on floor	Balance/partial motion	Full motion

	BEGINNER	INTERMEDIATE	ADVANCED

Stability ball reverse crunches

1 set

30 seconds

Knees to chest	Lift hips	Pause

Medicine ball toe touches

1 set

30 seconds

Knees bent	Arms extended	Heavier ball

REST 30 seconds

TRI-SET 2

		INTERMEDIATE	ADVANCED
Stability ball over/under crunch 1 set 45 seconds	Half rep	Full motion	Lift hips
Seated med ball Russian twists 1 set 30 seconds	Hands close to body	Arms extended	Heavier ball (or elevate feet)

	BEGINNER	INTERMEDIATE	ADVANCED
Stability ball knee-ins **1 set** **30 seconds**	Slow, ball under knees	Extend legs	Pike

REST 30 seconds | repeat cycle 1X | repeat cycle 2x | repeat cycle 3x

Week **4** Day **4**: Upper Body Strength Circuit

10-minute light cardiovascular warm up such as walking or stationary bike.

CIRCUIT

		INTERMEDIATE	ADVANCED

1-arm row

1 set

15 reps

 Light DB Medium DB Heavy DB

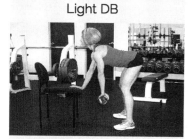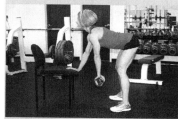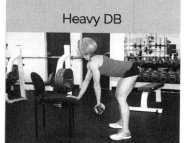

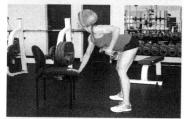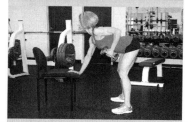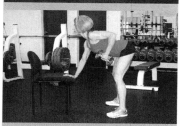

Rear lateral

1 set

15 reps

Light DB Medium DB Heavy DB

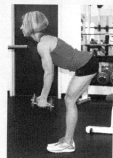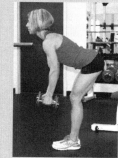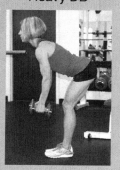

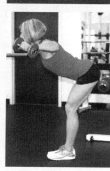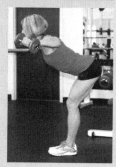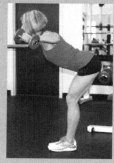

Stability ball chest press

1 set

15 reps

Stability ball fly

1 set

15 reps

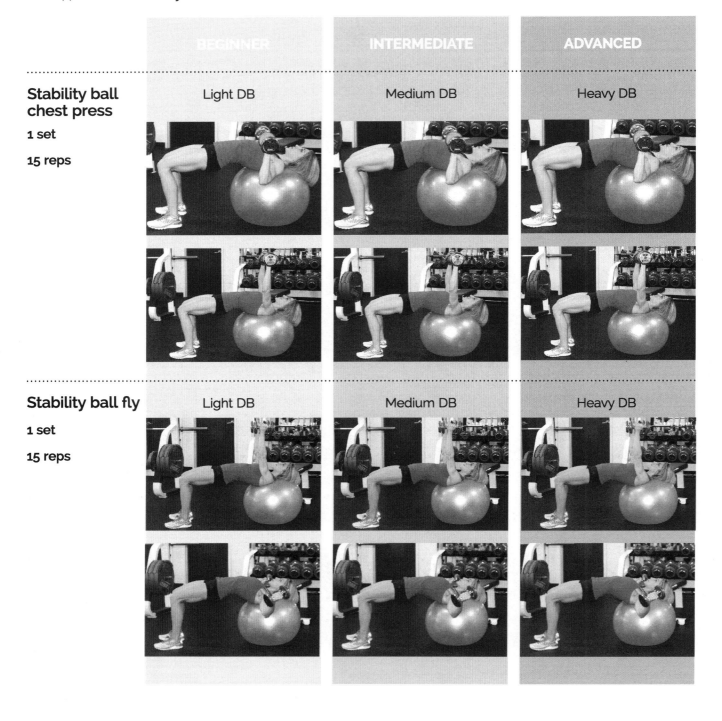

BEGINNER	INTERMEDIATE	ADVANCED
Light DB	Medium DB	Heavy DB
Light DB	Medium DB	Heavy DB

	INTERMEDIATE	ADVANCED
Overhead tricep extension 1 set 15 reps	Light DB	Medium DB	Heavy DB

Bicep curl 1 set 15 reps	Light DB	Medium DB	Heavy DB

REST 60 seconds

repeat cycle 3X	repeat cycle 4x	repeat cycle 5x

INCREASE WEIGHT PER ROUND AS TOLERATED

Week 4 Day 5: Lower Body Functional Training

10-minute light cardiovascular warm up such as walking or stationary bike.

CIRCUIT 1

	BEGINNER	INTERMEDIATE	ADVANCED
Jump rope 1 set 60 seconds	Simulated (no rope)	Full motion	Full motion
Body-weight squats 1 set 60 seconds	Hands at sides	Hands behind head	Hands up and back

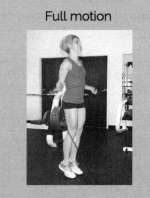

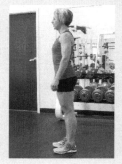

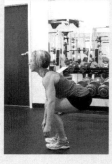

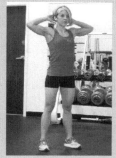

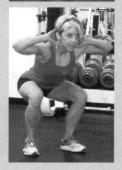

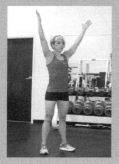

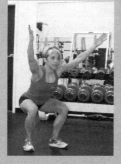

	INTERMEDIATE	ADVANCED

Side lunges

1 set

60 seconds

Step out	Half lunge	Full lunge

	BEGINNER	INTERMEDIATE	ADVANCED
Push up plank spidermans **1 set** **45 seconds**	Standing 	On knees 	Full motion

REST 30 seconds

CIRCUIT 2

		INTERMEDIATE	ADVANCED

Jump rope

1 set

60 seconds

Simulated (no rope)	Full motion	Full motion

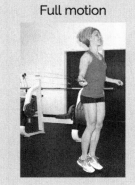
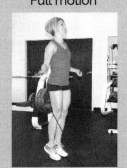

Sumo squat

1 set

60 seconds

Partial squat	Half squat	Full squat

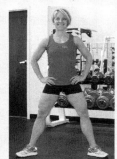
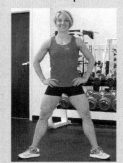
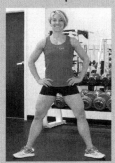

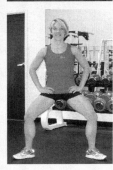
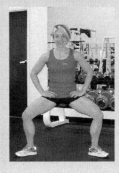
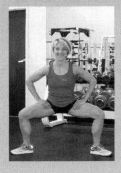

	BEGINNER	INTERMEDIATE	ADVANCED

Alternating lunges

1 set

60 seconds

Partial lunge	Half lunge	Full lunge

Pushup plank lateral hops

1 set

60 seconds

Plank only	Step out	Full motion

REST 30 seconds

repeat cycle 3X	repeat cycle 4x	repeat cycle 5x

Week 4 Day 6: High-Intensity Interval Cardio & Abs

10-minute light cardiovascular warm up such as walking or stationary bike; stretch legs lightly.

- A circuit of cardio intervals will be superset with abdominal exercises.

- You may use cardio form such as jogging, elliptical, or bike.

- As intervals shorten, intensity should increase.

CIRCUIT

		INTERMEDIATE	ADVANCED
Cardio interval 1 set: 60 sec.	Bike	Elliptical	Jog or functional movement
Med ball mountain climbers 1 set 60 seconds	Plank	Knees to chest	Full motion

	BEGINNER	INTERMEDIATE	ADVANCED
Cardio interval **1 set: 45 sec.**	Bike	Elliptical	Jog or functional movement
Med ball spidermans **1 set** **60 seconds**	Plank 	Knees out 	Add pushup
Cardio interval **1 set: 30 sec.**	Bike	Elliptical	Jog or functional movement
Cross-body mountain climbers **1 set** **60 seconds**	Plank 	Knees cross 	Full motion

		INTERMEDIATE	ADVANCED
Cardio interval 1 set: 15 sec.	Bike	Elliptical	Jog or functional movement
Med ball twist & kick 1 set 60 seconds	Plank	No kick	Full motion

REST 60 seconds

repeat cycle 1X   repeat cycle 2x   repeat cycle 3x

Week 5 Day 1: Upper Body Functional Training

10-minute light cardiovascular warm up such as walking or stationary bike.

GIANT SET 1

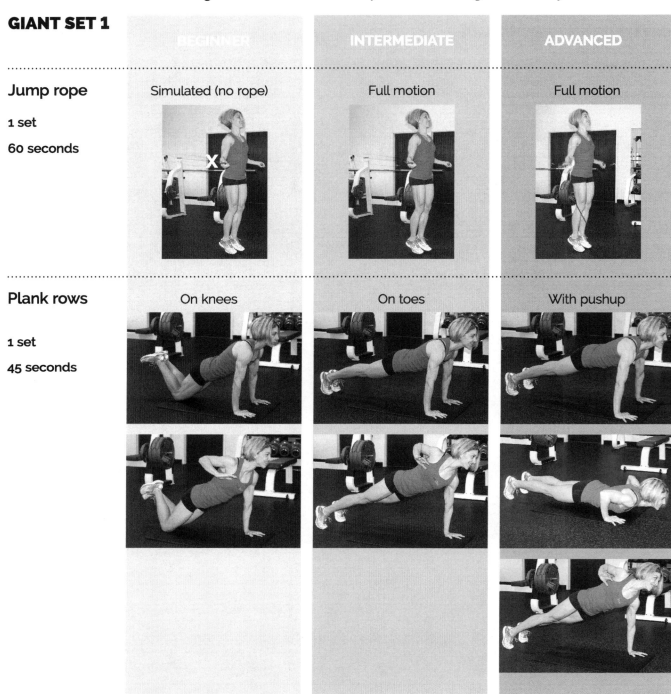

	BEGINNER	INTERMEDIATE	ADVANCED
Jump rope 1 set 60 seconds	Simulated (no rope)	Full motion	Full motion
Plank rows 1 set 45 seconds	On knees	On toes	With pushup

Pushups

1 set

45 seconds

BEGINNER	INTERMEDIATE	ADVANCED
Against wall	On knees	On toes

Good mornings

1 set

30 seconds

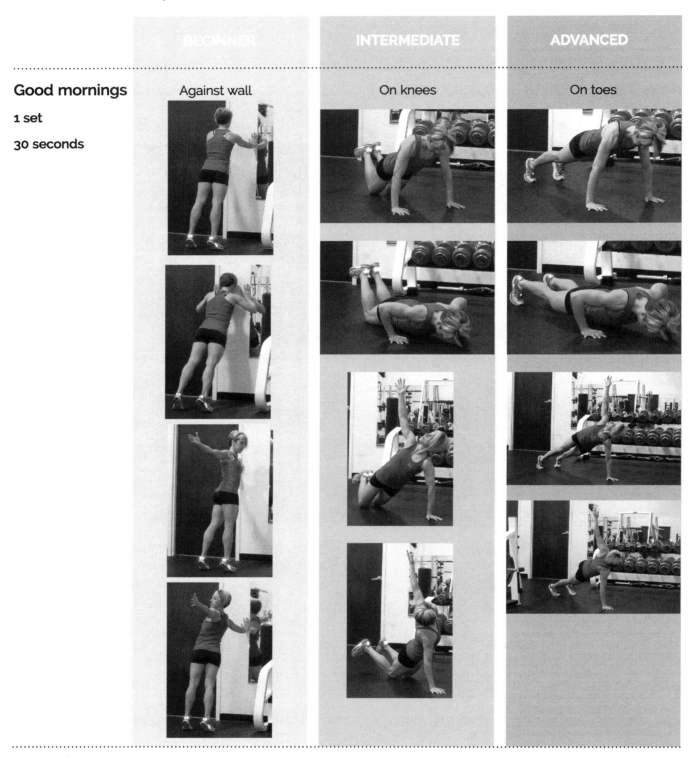

BEGINNER	INTERMEDIATE	ADVANCED
Against wall	On knees	On toes

REST 30 seconds

GIANT SET 2

		INTERMEDIATE	ADVANCED

Jump rope

1 set

60 seconds

Simulated (no rope)	Full motion	Full motion
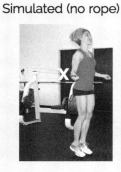	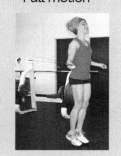	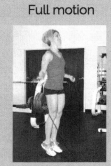

Tricep band kickbacks

1 set

45 seconds

Light resistance	Medium resistance	Heavy resistance
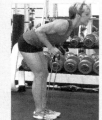 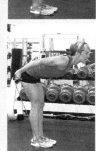	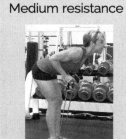 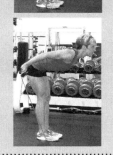	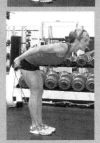

Bicep band curls

1 set

45 seconds

Light resistance	Medium resistance	Heavy resistance
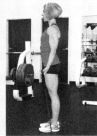 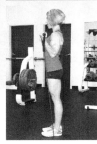	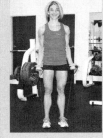 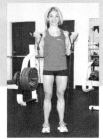	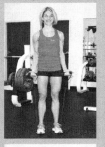 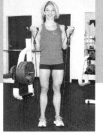

	BEGINNER	INTERMEDIATE	ADVANCED
Burpees **1 set** **30 seconds**	Walk through	Full motion	With pushup

REST 30 seconds

repeat cycle 2X	repeat cycle 3x	repeat cycle 4x

Week 5 Day 2: Lower Body Strength Circuit

10-minute light cardiovascular warm up such as walking or stationary bike.

SUPERSET 1

		INTERMEDIATE	ADVANCED
Squats	Half squat	Full squat	DB squat
1 set			
20 reps			

Stiff-legged dead lift	No weight	Light DBs	Medium DBs
1 set			
20 reps			

REST 30 seconds

SUPERSET 2

	BEGINNER	INTERMEDIATE	ADVANCED

Step-ups

1 set

20 reps

No weight	Light DBs	Medium DBs

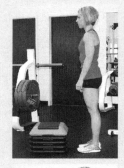
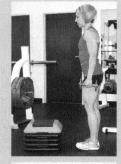
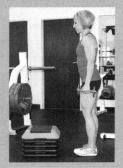

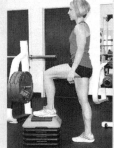
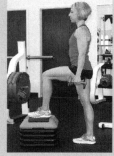
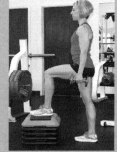

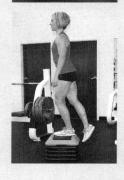
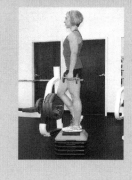
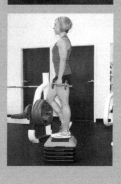

	INTERMEDIATE	ADVANCED

Stability ball hamstring curl

1 set

20 reps

Curl only	Curl and contract	Curl and bridge
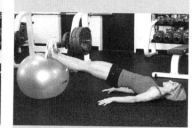	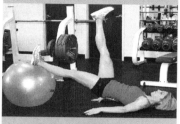	
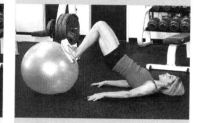	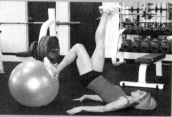	

REST 30 seconds

SUPERSET 3

Goblet squats
1 set

20 reps

Half squat	Full squat	DB squat
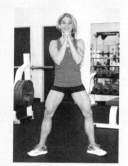	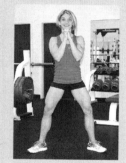	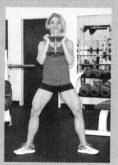
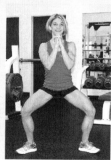	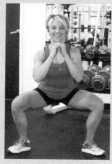	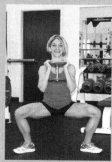

Band hamstring curl

1 set

20 reps

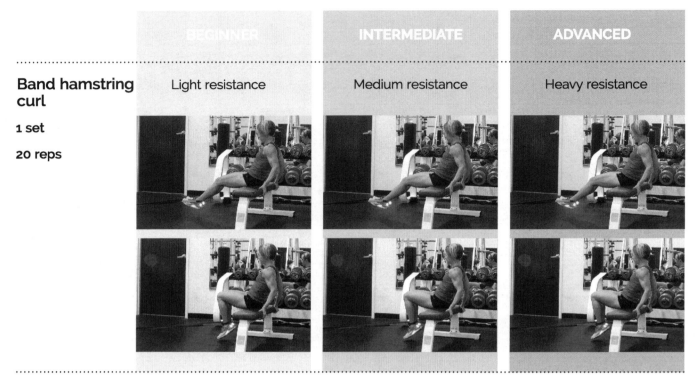

BEGINNER	INTERMEDIATE	ADVANCED
Light resistance	Medium resistance	Heavy resistance

REST 30 seconds

repeat cycle 2X   repeat cycle 3x   repeat cycle 4x

INCREASE WEIGHT PER ROUND AS TOLERATED

Week 5 Day 3: Steady-State Cardio & Abs

10-minute light cardiovascular warm up such as walking or stationary bike; stretch legs lightly.

TRI-SET 1

		INTERMEDIATE	ADVANCED
Cardio interval 1 set: 10 min.	55 percent max HR	60 percent max HR	65 percent max HR
V-ups 1 set 60 seconds	Hands on floor	Balance/partial motion	Full motion
Bicycle crunches 1 set 30 seconds	Slow, knees bent	Extend leg	Pause

REST 30 seconds

TRI-SET 2

	BEGINNER	INTERMEDIATE	ADVANCED
Cardio interval 1 set: 10 min.	60 percent max HR	65 percent max HR	70 percent max HR
Reverse crunches 1 set 60 seconds	Knees to chest	Lift hips	Pause
Bicycle crunches 1 set 30 seconds	Slow, knees bent	Extend legs	Pause

REST 45 seconds

TRI-SET 3

		INTERMEDIATE	ADVANCED
Cardio interval 1 set: 10 min.	65 percent max HR	70 percent max HR	75 percent max HR
Supermans 1 set 60 seconds	Alternate arms/legs	Quadriped	Prone-arms/legs together

	Prone	On stability ball	Arms Out
Hyperextensions 1 set 30 seconds			

REST 60 seconds

REPEAT ALL CORE EXERCISES 1 TIME IN SUCCESSION FOR 30 SECONDS TO FINISH WORKOUT.

Week 5 Day 4: Upper Body Strength Circuit

10-minute light cardiovascular warm up such as walking or stationary bike.

SUPERSET 1

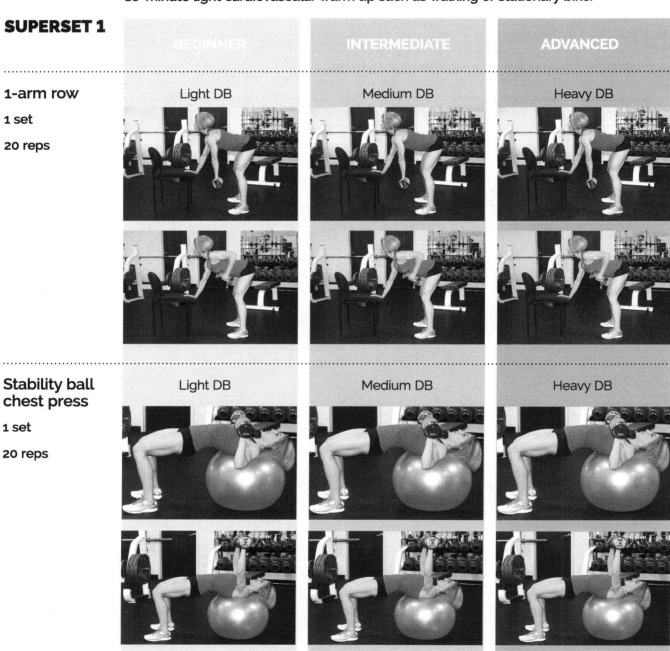

	BEGINNER	INTERMEDIATE	ADVANCED
1-arm row 1 set 20 reps	Light DB	Medium DB	Heavy DB
Stability ball chest press 1 set 20 reps	Light DB	Medium DB	Heavy DB

REST 30 seconds

SUPERSET 2

		INTERMEDIATE	ADVANCED

Rear lateral

1 set

20 reps

Light DB	Medium DB	Heavy DB

Stability ball fly

1 set

20 reps

Light DB	Medium DB	Heavy DB

REST 30 seconds

SUPERSET 3

	BEGINNER	INTERMEDIATE	ADVANCED
Shoulder lateral 1 set 20 reps	Light DB	Medium DB	Heavy DB
Overhead press 1 set 20 reps	Light DB	Medium DB	Heavy DB

REST 30 seconds

SUPERSET 4

	BEGINNER	INTERMEDIATE	ADVANCED

Overhead tricep extension

1 set

20 reps

Light DB	Medium DB	Heavy DB

Bicep curl

1 set

20 reps

Light DB	Medium DB	Heavy DB

REST 30 seconds

repeat cycle 2X	repeat cycle 3x	repeat cycle 4x

INCREASE WEIGHT PER ROUND AS TOLERATED

Week 5 Day 5: Lower Body Functional Training

10-minute light cardiovascular warm up such as walking or stationary bike.

CIRCUIT 1

	BEGINNER	INTERMEDIATE	ADVANCED
Jump rope 1 set 60 seconds	Simulated (no rope)	Full motion	Full motion
Body-weight squats 1 set 45 seconds	Hands at sides	Hands behind head	Hands up and back

		INTERMEDIATE	ADVANCED

Sumo squat

1 set

45 seconds

Partial squat	Half squat	Full squat

	BEGINNER	INTERMEDIATE	ADVANCED
Pushup plank twist & kick **1 set** **30 seconds**	Standing	No kick	Full motion

REST 30 seconds

CIRCUIT 2

		INTERMEDIATE	ADVANCED
Jump rope 1 set 60 seconds	Simulated (no rope)	Full motion	Full motion
Side lunges 1 set 45 seconds	Step out	Half lunge	Full lunge

	BEGINNER	INTERMEDIATE	ADVANCED

Alternating lunges

1 set

45 seconds

Partial lunge	Half lunge	Full lunge

Pushup plank ski hops

1 set

30 seconds

Plank only	Walk through	Full motion

REST 30 seconds

repeat cycle 2X | repeat cycle 3x | repeat cycle 4x

Week 5 Day 6: High-Intensity Interval Cardio & Abs

10-minute light cardiovascular warm up such as walking or stationary bike; stretch legs lightly.

- A circuit of cardio intervals will be superset with abdominal exercises.
- You may use cardio form such as jogging, elliptical, or bike.
- As intervals shorten, intensity should increase.

SUPERSET 1

		INTERMEDIATE	ADVANCED
Cardio interval 1 set: 60 sec.	Bike	Elliptical	Jog or functional movement
Med ball mountain climbers 1 set 60 seconds	Plank	Knees to chest	Full motion

SUPERSET 2

	BEGINNER	INTERMEDIATE	ADVANCED
Cardio interval 1 set: 60 sec.	Bike	Elliptical	Jog or functional movement
Med ball spidermans 1 set 60 seconds	Plank	Knees out	Add pushup

SUPERSET 3

	BEGINNER	INTERMEDIATE	ADVANCED
Cardio interval 2 sets: 30 sec.	Bike	Elliptical	Jog or functional movement
Cross-body mountain climbers 2 sets 60 seconds	Plank	Knees cross	Full motion

SUPERSET 4

	BEGINNER	INTERMEDIATE	ADVANCED
Cardio interval 3 sets: 15 sec.	Bike	Elliptical	Jog or functional movement
Med ball twist & kick 3 sets 60 seconds	Plank	No kick	Full motion

REST 60 seconds

repeat cycle 1X   repeat cycle 2x   repeat cycle 3x

Week 6 Day 1: Upper Body Functional Training

10-minute light cardiovascular warm up such as walking or stationary bike.

GIANT SET 1

	BEGINNER	INTERMEDIATE	ADVANCED
Jump rope 1 set 60 seconds	Simulated (no rope)	Full motion	Full motion
Plank rows 1 set 60 seconds	On knees	On toes	With pushup

Pushups

1 set

60 seconds

BEGINNER

INTERMEDIATE

ADVANCED

Against wall

On knees

On toes

Good mornings

1 set

45 seconds

BEGINNER	INTERMEDIATE	ADVANCED
Against wall	On knees	On toes

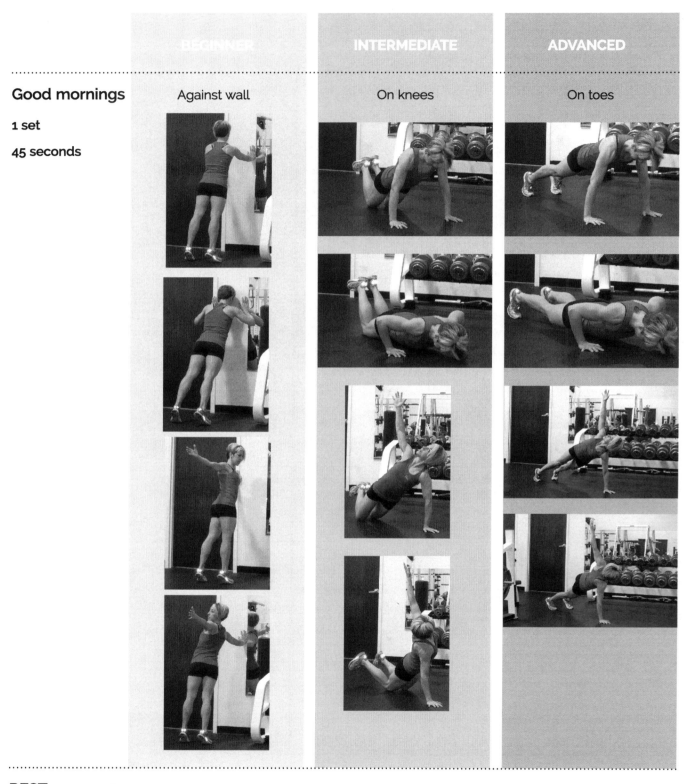

REST 30 seconds

GIANT SET 2

	BEGINNER	INTERMEDIATE	ADVANCED

Jump rope
1 set

60 seconds

Simulated (no rope)	Full motion	Full motion

Tricep band kickbacks
1 set

60 seconds

Light resistance	Medium resistance	Heavy resistance

Bicep band curls
1 set

60 seconds

Light resistance	Medium resistance	Heavy resistance

	BEGINNER	INTERMEDIATE	ADVANCED
Burpees **1 set** **45 seconds**	Walk through 	Full motion 	With pushup

REST 30 seconds   repeat cycle 3X   repeat cycle 4x   repeat cycle 5x

Week 6 Day 2: Lower Body Strength Circuit

10-minute light cardiovascular warm up such as walking or stationary bike.

SUPERSET 1

	BEGINNER	INTERMEDIATE	ADVANCED

Squats

1 set

15 reps

Half squat	Full squat	DB squat

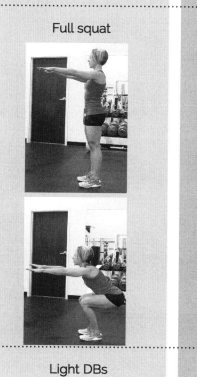
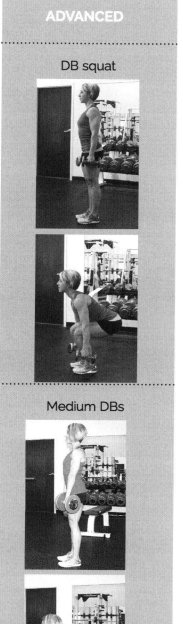

Stiff-legged dead lift

1 set

15 reps

No weight	Light DBs	Medium DBs

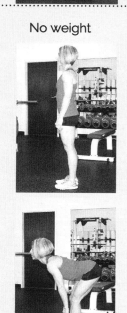
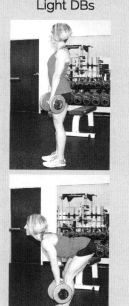
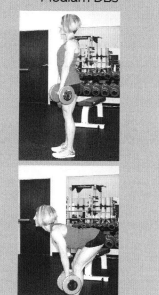

REST 30 seconds

SUPERSET 2

	BEGINNER	INTERMEDIATE	ADVANCED

Step-ups

1 set

15 reps

No weight	Light DBs	Medium DBs
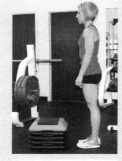	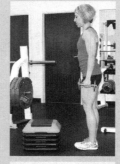	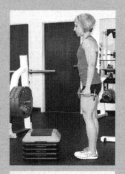
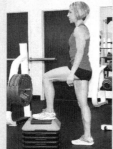	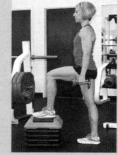	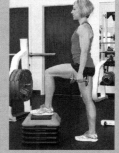
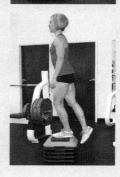	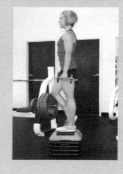	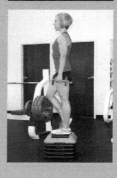

	INTERMEDIATE	ADVANCED

Stability ball hamstring curl

1 set

15 reps

Curl only	Curl and contract	Curl and bridge

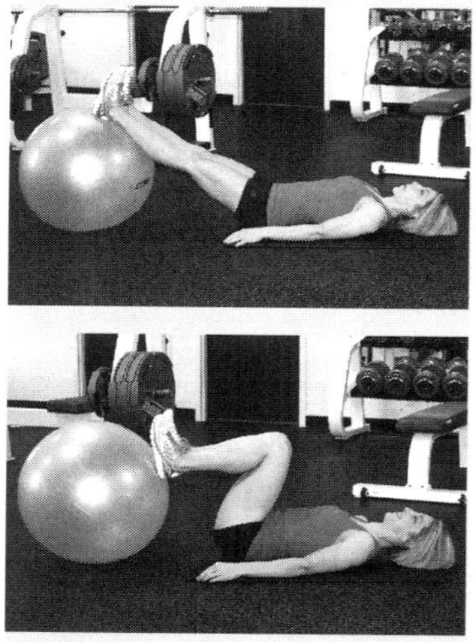

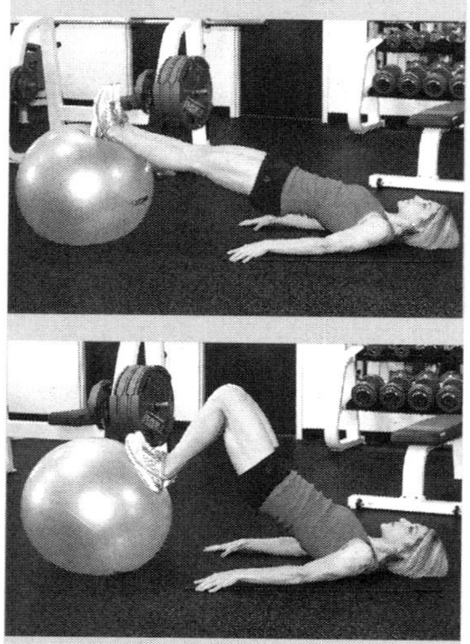

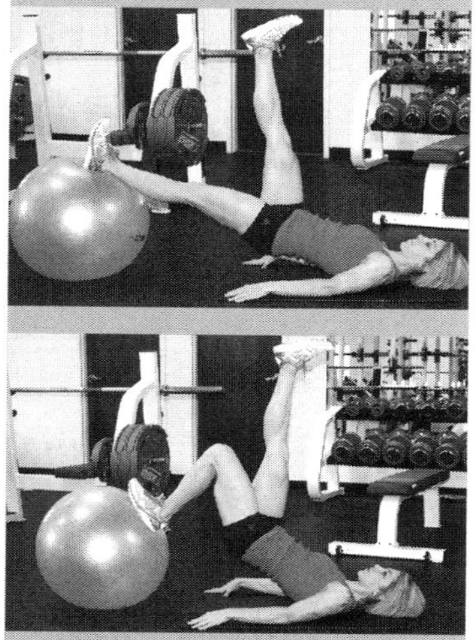

REST 30 seconds

SUPERSET 3

Goblet squats

1 set

15 reps

Half squat	Full squat	DB squat

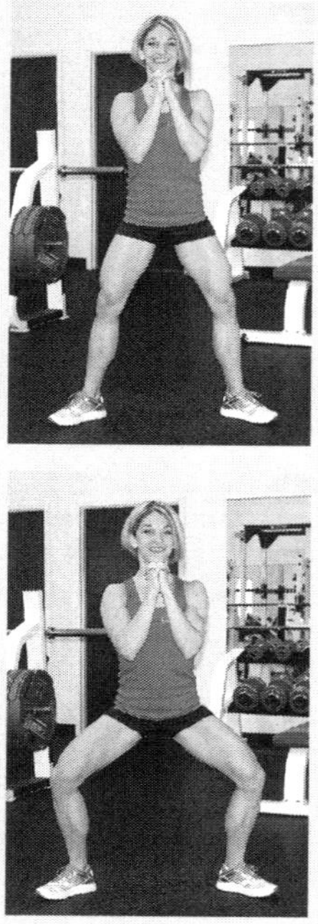

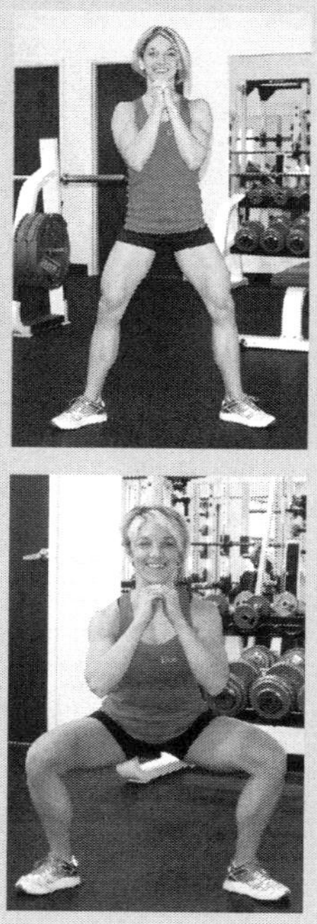

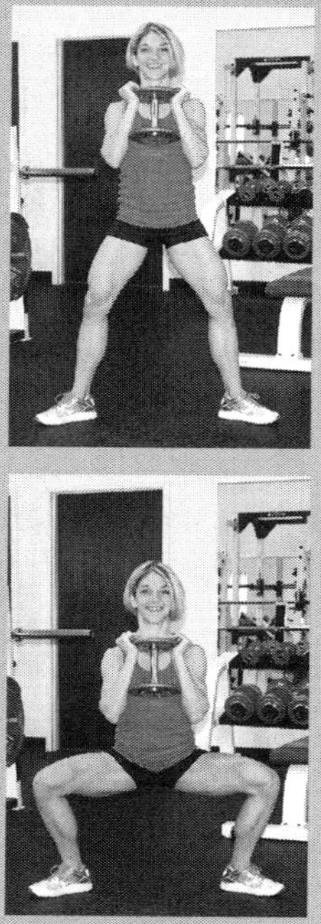

Band hamstring curl

1 set

15 reps

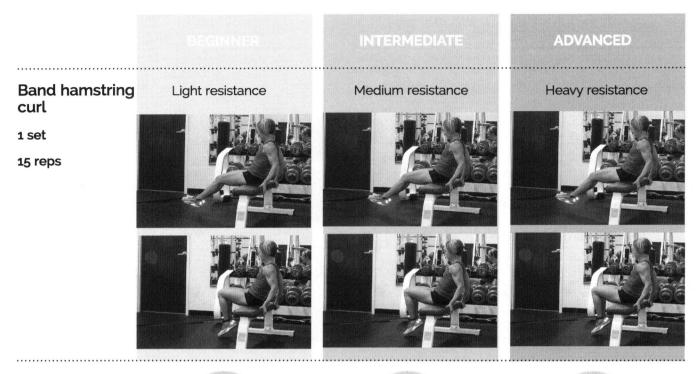

BEGINNER	INTERMEDIATE	ADVANCED
Light resistance	Medium resistance	Heavy resistance

REST 30 seconds

repeat cycle 3X   repeat cycle 4x   repeat cycle 5x

INCREASE WEIGHT PER ROUND AS TOLERATED

Week 6 Day 3: Steady-State Cardio & Abs

10-minute light cardiovascular warm up such as walking or stationary bike.

Cardio intervals with abdominal exercises: perform all three sets of ab exercises in a row, with 15 seconds of rest between sets.

SUPERSET 1

		INTERMEDIATE	ADVANCED
Cardio interval 1 set: 15 min.	60 percent max HR	65 percent max HR	70 percent max HR
Reverse crunches 1 set: 60, 40, 20 sec.	Knees to chest	Lift hips	Pause

REST 60 seconds

SUPERSET 2

	BEGINNER	INTERMEDIATE	ADVANCED
Cardio interval **1 set: 10 min.**	65 percent max HR	70 percent max HR	75 percent max HR
Crunches **3 sets: 60, 40, 20 sec.**	Knees bent	Pause	Add reach

REST 60 seconds

SUPERSET 3

		INTERMEDIATE	ADVANCED
Cardio interval 1 set: 5 min.	70 percent max HR	75 percent max HR	80 percent max HR
Standing Russian twists 3 sets 60, 40, 20 sec.	Hands close to body	Arms extended	Heavier band

REST 60 seconds

REPEAT ALL FOUR ABDOMINAL EXERCISES IN A ROW FOR 30 SECONDS EACH.

Week 6 Day 4: Upper Body Strength Circuit

10-minute light cardiovascular warm up such as walking or stationary bike.

SUPERSET 1

	BEGINNER	INTERMEDIATE	ADVANCED
1-arm row 1 set 15 reps	Light DB 	Medium DB 	Heavy DB
Stability ball chest press 1 set 15 reps	Light DB 	Medium DB 	Heavy DB

REST 30 seconds

SUPERSET 2

		INTERMEDIATE	ADVANCED

Rear lateral

1 set

15 reps

Light DB	Medium DB	Heavy DB

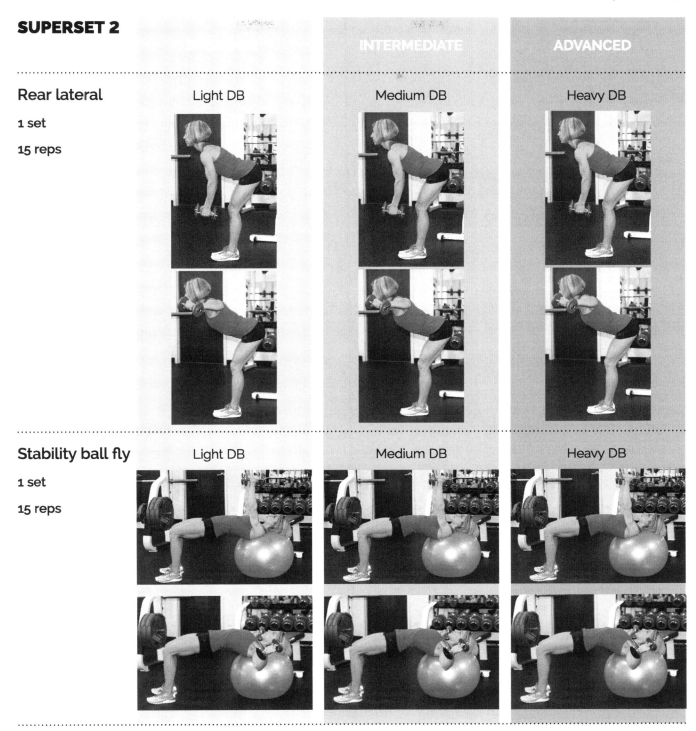

Stability ball fly

1 set

15 reps

Light DB	Medium DB	Heavy DB

REST 30 seconds

SUPERSET 3

	BEGINNER	INTERMEDIATE	ADVANCED
Shoulder lateral 1 set 15 reps	Light DB 	Medium DB 	Heavy DB
Overhead press 1 set 15 reps	Light DB 	Medium DB 	Heavy DB

REST 30 seconds

SUPERSET 4

	Light DB	INTERMEDIATE Medium DB	ADVANCED Heavy DB
Overhead tricep extension **1 set** 15 reps			
Bicep curl **1 set** 15 reps	Light DB	Medium DB	Heavy DB

REST 30 seconds	repeat cycle 3x	repeat cycle 4x	repeat cycle 5x

INCREASE WEIGHT PER ROUND AS TOLERATED

Week 6 Day 5: Lower Body Functional Training

10-minute light cardiovascular warm up such as walking or stationary bike.

CIRCUIT 1

	BEGINNER	INTERMEDIATE	ADVANCED
Jump rope 1 set 60 seconds	Simulated (no rope)	Full motion	Full motion
	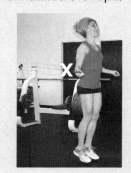	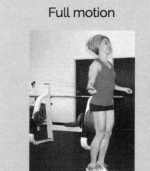	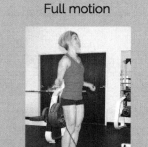
Body-weight squats 1 set 60 seconds	Hands at sides	Hands behind head	Hands up and back
	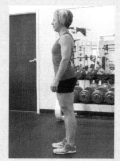 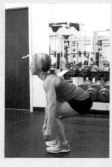	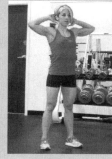 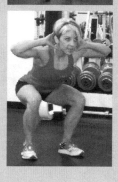	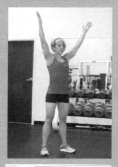 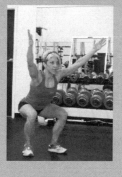

Sumo squat

1 set

60 seconds

BEGINNER	INTERMEDIATE	ADVANCED
Partial squat	Half squat	Full squat

	BEGINNER	INTERMEDIATE	ADVANCED
Pushup plank twist & kick **1 set** **45 seconds**	Standing	Knees only	Full motion

REST 30 seconds

CIRCUIT 2

		INTERMEDIATE	ADVANCED

Jump rope

1 set

60 seconds

Simulated (no rope)	Full motion	Full motion
	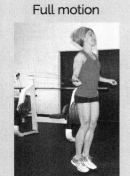	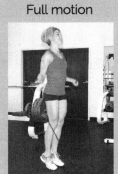

Side lunges

1 set

60 seconds

Step out	Half lunge	Full lunge
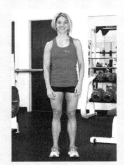	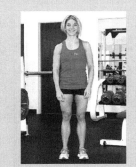	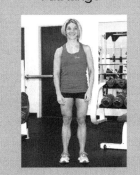
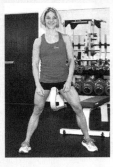	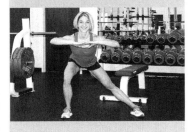	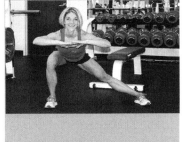

	BEGINNER	INTERMEDIATE	ADVANCED

Alternating lunges

1 set

60 seconds

Partial lunge	Half lunge	Full lunge

Pushup plank ski hops

1 set

45 seconds

Plank only	Walk through	Full motion

REST 30 seconds

repeat cycle 3x	repeat cycle 4x	repeat cycle 5x

Week 6 Day 6: High-Intensity Interval Cardio & Abs

10-minute light cardiovascular warm up such as walking or stationary bike; stretch legs lightly.

- You may use any cardio form such as jogging, elliptical, or bike.
- Maximum heart rate equals 220 minus your age.
- Active rest example: walk.

CIRCUIT		INTERMEDIATE	ADVANCED
Interval 1 1 set: 4 min.	55 percent max HR	60 percent max HR	65 percent max HR
Stability ball crunches 1 set 60 seconds	Hands behind head	Higher on ball	Hold med ball
Interval 2 1 set: 3 min.	60 percent max HR	65 percent max HR	70 percent max HR

	BEGINNER	INTERMEDIATE	ADVANCED
Stability ball reverse crunches 1 set 60 seconds	Knees to chest 	Lift hips 	Lift and pause
Interval 3 1 set: 2 min.	65 percent max HR	70 percent max HR	75 percent max HR
Stability ball Russian twists 1 set 60 seconds	Use hands to balance 	Arms extended 	Hold med ball

		INTERMEDIATE	ADVANCED
Interval 4 2 set: 1 min.	70 percent max HR	75 percent max HR	80 percent max HR
Stability ball roll-outs 2 sets 60 seconds	On elbows 	Extend arms slightly 	Pike back and forth
Interval 5 3 sets: 30 sec.	75 percent max HR	80 percent max HR	85 percent max HR
Stability ball planks 3 sets 45 seconds	On knees 	On toes 	Full extension

Week 7 Day 1: Upper Body Functional Training

10-minute light cardiovascular warm up such as walking or stationary bike.

CIRCUIT	BEGINNER	INTERMEDIATE	ADVANCED
Jump rope 1 set 60 seconds	Simulated (no rope)	Full motion	Full motion
Plank rows 1 set 45 seconds	On knees	On toes	With pushup

		INTERMEDIATE	ADVANCED

Band pull-through

1 set

45 seconds

Light resistance	Medium resistance	Heavy resistance

Mountain climber

1 set

30 seconds

Standing	Walk through	Full motion

	BEGINNER	INTERMEDIATE	ADVANCED

Pushups

1 set

45 seconds

Against wall	On knees	On toes

Band fly

1 set

45 seconds

Light resistance	Medium resistance	Heavy resistance

		INTERMEDIATE	**ADVANCED**

Pushup plank lateral hops

1 set

30 seconds

On knees/lateral taps

On toes/feet apart

On toes/feet together

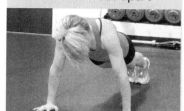
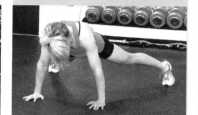
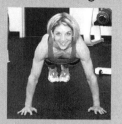
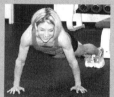
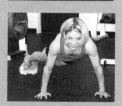

Bicep band curls

1 set

45 seconds

Light resistance

Medium resistance

Heavy resistance

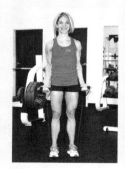
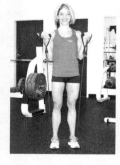
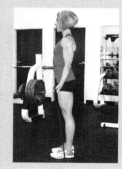
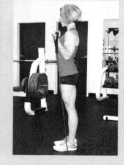
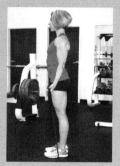
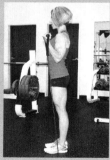

	BEGINNER	INTERMEDIATE	ADVANCED
Tricep band kickbacks **1 set** **45 seconds**	Light resistance 	Medium resistance 	Heavy resistance

Burpees

1 set

30 seconds

Walk through	INTERMEDIATE	ADVANCED
	Full motion	With pushup

REST 60 seconds

repeat cycle 3x · repeat cycle 4x · repeat cycle 5x

Week 7 Day 2: Lower Body Strength Circuit

10-minute light cardiovascular warm up such as walking or stationary bike.

SUPERSET 1

	BEGINNER	INTERMEDIATE	ADVANCED
Squats.	Half squat	Full squat	DB squat

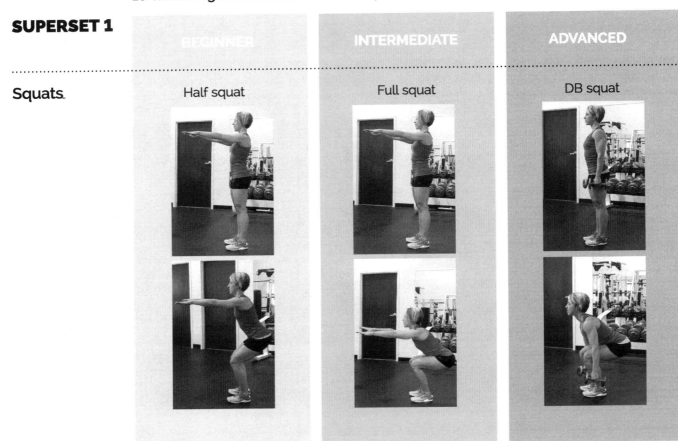

Step-ups

1 set

15 reps

INTERMEDIATE

ADVANCED

No weight

Light DBs

Medium DBs

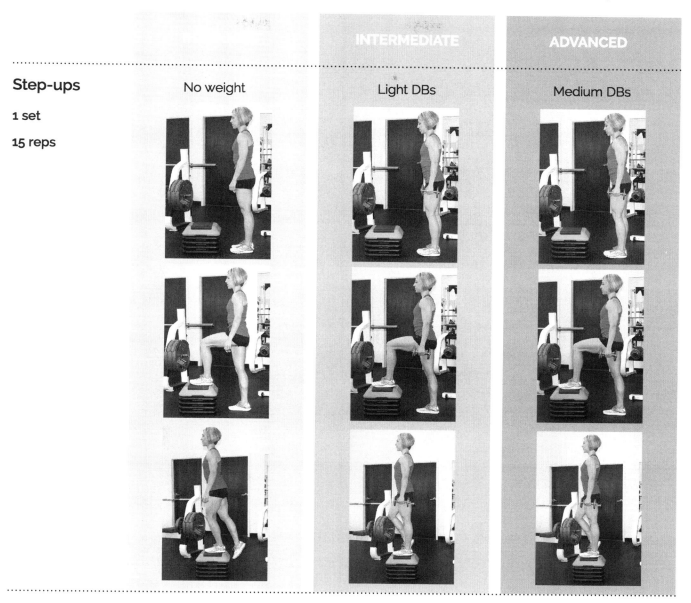

REST 30 seconds

SUPERSET 2

	BEGINNER	INTERMEDIATE	ADVANCED

Goblet squats

1 set

15 reps

Half squat

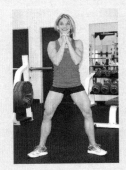

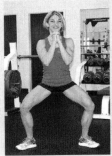

Full squat

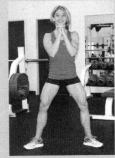

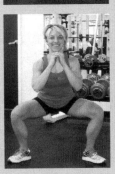

DB squat

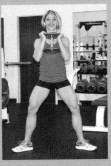

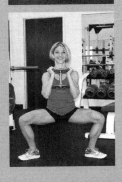

DB walking lunges

1 set

15 reps

No weight	INTERMEDIATE	ADVANCED
	Light DBs	Medium DBs

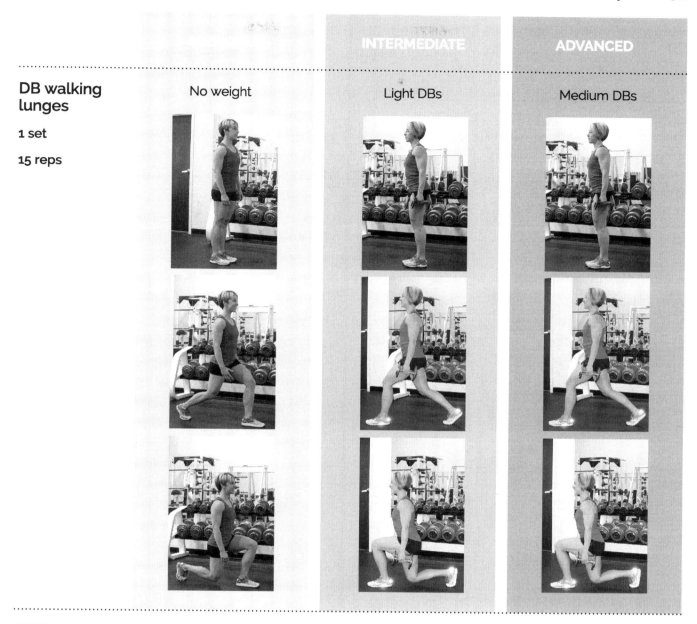

REST 30 seconds

SUPERSET 3

	BEGINNER	INTERMEDIATE	ADVANCED
Stiff-legged dead lift **1 set** **15 reps**	No weight	Light DBs	Medium DBs
Stability ball hamstring curl **1 set** **15 reps**	Curl only	Curl and contract	Curl and bridge

REST 30 seconds

SUPERSET 4

		INTERMEDIATE	**ADVANCED**

Calf raise

1 set

15 reps

No weight	Light DBs	Medium DBs

Band hamstring curl

1 set

15 reps

Light resistance	Medium resistance	Heavy resistance

REST 30 seconds

repeat cycle 3x	repeat cycle 4x	repeat cycle 5x

INCREASE WEIGHT PER ROUND AS TOLERATED

Week 7 Day 3: Steady-State Cardio & Abs

10-minute light cardiovascular warm up such as walking or stationary bike.

CARDIO INTERVALS

	BEGINNER	INTERMEDIATE	ADVANCED
Cardio interval **1 set: 20 min.**	55 percent max HR	60 percent max HR	65 percent max HR
Stretch break 2 minutes			
Cardio interval **1 set: 15 min.**	60 percent max HR	65 percent max HR	70 percent max HR
Stretch break 2 minutes			
Cardio interval **1 set: 10 min.**	65 percent max HR	70 percent max HR	75 percent max HR
Stretch break 2 minutes			

CORE CIRCUIT

	Walk through	INTERMEDIATE	ADVANCED
		Full motion	Increase speed

Med ball mountain climers

1 set

30 seconds

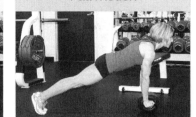
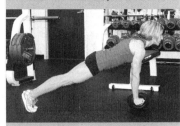
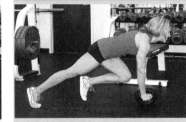
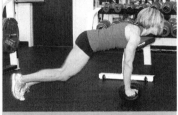
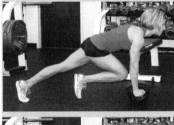
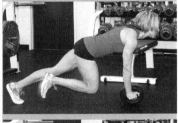
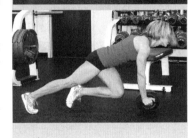
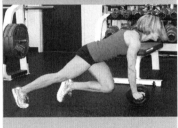

V-ups

1 set

30 seconds

Plank

1 set

60 seconds

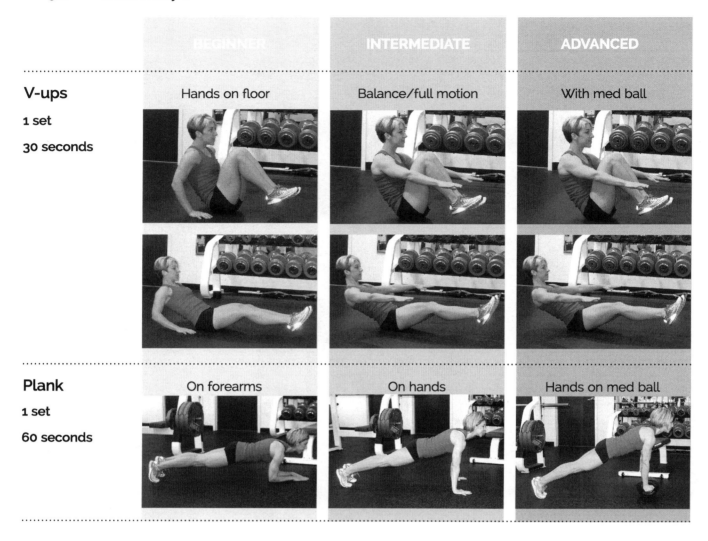

	BEGINNER	INTERMEDIATE	ADVANCED
V-ups	Hands on floor	Balance/full motion	With med ball
Plank	On forearms	On hands	Hands on med ball

repeat cycle 3x   repeat cycle 4x   repeat cycle 5x

Week 7 Day 4: Upper Body Strength Circuit

10-minute light cardiovascular warm up such as walking or stationary bike.

SUPERSET 1

		INTERMEDIATE	ADVANCED

1-arm row

1 set

15 reps

Light DB	Medium DB	Heavy DB

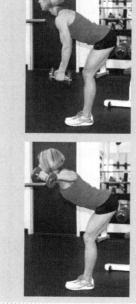

Rear lateral

1 set

15 reps

Light DB	Medium DB	Heavy DB

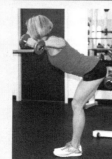 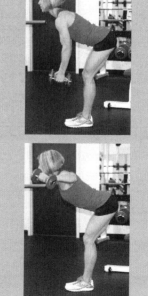

REST 30 seconds

SUPERSET 2

	BEGINNER	INTERMEDIATE	ADVANCED
Stability ball chest press **1 set** **15 reps**	Light DB	Medium DB	Heavy DB
Stability ball fly **1 set** **15 reps**	Light DB	Medium DB	Heavy DB

REST 30 seconds

SUPERSET 3

		INTERMEDIATE	ADVANCED

Shoulder lateral

1 set

15 reps

Light DB	Medium DB	Heavy DB

Overhead press

1 set

15 reps

Light DB	Medium DB	Heavy DB

REST 30 seconds

SUPERSET 4

	BEGINNER	INTERMEDIATE	ADVANCED
Overhead tricep extension **1 set** **15 reps**	Light DB	Medium DB	Heavy DB
Tricep kickback **1 set** **15 reps**	Light DB	Medium DB	Heavy DB

REST 30 seconds

SUPERSET 5

		INTERMEDIATE	ADVANCED

Bicep curl

1 set

15 reps

Light DB Medium DB Heavy DB

Bicep hammer curl

1 set

15 reps

Light DB Medium DB Heavy DB

REST 30 seconds

repeat cycle 3x repeat cycle 4x repeat cycle 5x

INCREASE WEIGHT PER ROUND AS TOLERATED

Week 7 Day 5: Lower Body Functional Training

10-minute light cardiovascular warm up such as walking or stationary bike.

CIRCUIT

	BEGINNER	INTERMEDIATE	ADVANCED
Jump rope 1 set 60 seconds	Simulated (no rope)	Full motion	Full motion
		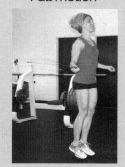	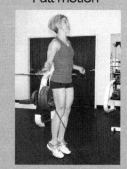
Body-weight squats 1 set 45 seconds	Hands at sides	Hands behind head	Hands up and back
	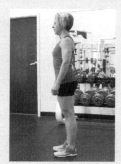 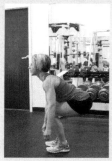	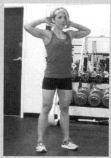 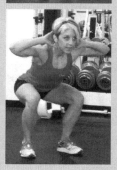	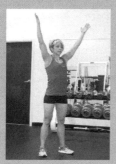 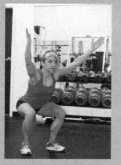

		INTERMEDIATE	ADVANCED
Side lunges 1 set 45 seconds	Step out	Half lunge	Full lunge

	Half kicks	Full kicks	Squat kicks
Alternating front kicks 1 set 30 seconds			

	BEGINNER	INTERMEDIATE	ADVANCED

Sumo squat

1 set

45 seconds

Partial squat	Half squat	Full squat

Alternating lunges

1 set

45 seconds

Partial lunge	Half lunge	Full lunge

Flying hop kick

1 set

30 seconds

Knee up/half kick	INTERMEDIATE Knee up/full kick	ADVANCED Full motion

REST 60 seconds

repeat cycle 3x   repeat cycle 4x   repeat cycle 5x

Week 7 Day 6: High-Intensity Interval Cardio & Abs

10-minute light cardiovascular warm up such as walking or stationary bike; stretch legs lightly.

You may use any cardio form such as jogging, elliptical, or bike.

Maximum heart rate equals 220 minus your age.

Active rest example: walk.

CIRCUIT	BEGINNER	INTERMEDIATE	ADVANCED
Interval 1 1 set: 5 min.	55 percent max HR	60 percent max HR	65 percent max HR
Active rest 1 set: 60 sec.			
Interval 2 1 set: 4 min.	60 percent max HR	65 percent max HR	70 percent max HR
Active rest 1 set: 60 sec.			
Interval 3 1 set: 4 min.	65 percent max HR	70 percent max HR	75 percent max HR

		INTERMEDIATE	ADVANCED
Stability ball knee-ins 1 set 60 seconds	Half rep	Knees to chest	Pike
Interval 4 2 sets: 2 min.	70 percent max HR	75 percent max HR	80 percent max HR
Stability ball reverse crunches 1 set 60 seconds	Knees to chest	Lift hips	Pause
Interval 5 3 sets: 1 min.	75 percent max HR	80 percent max HR	85 percent max HR

	BEGINNER	INTERMEDIATE	ADVANCED
Stability ball over-unders 3 sets 60 seconds	Bent knees 	Full motion 	Lift hips
Interval 6 4 sets: 30 seconds	80 percent max HR	85 percent max HR	90 percent max HR
Stability ball roll-outs 4 sets 45 seconds	On knees 	Extend arms slightly 	Pike back and forth

Week **8** Day **1**
DAY 50!

Congratulations, you made it through your first cycle! We hope that we've whetted your appetite—pun intended—for more progress. You can repeat the plan exactly as you just performed it to gain more competence with form and to progress your fitness level, or you can advance through optional progressions. You can move up intensity levels (from beginner to intermediate) on some exercises, some days, or the entire plan. You can also expand your repertoire of exercises and move into substantial progressions on our website: thedietdoc.com. You'll find a video library of exercises and optional programs to challenge even the craziest athlete. Contact us from the site if you have any questions—we welcome your comments!

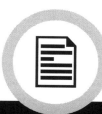

SECTION 7:
Appendices

Quick Recovery from Setbacks

For _____

Why I'm changing this behavior:

1. _____

2. _____

3. _____

My **Quick Recovery Plan** for managing _____

1. _____

2. _____

3. _____

4. _____

5. _____

Back–up Plan

If any lapses occur before _____ **I will:**

1. Think of the experience in a positive and constructive way and understand that a lapse is not a total relapse. I can take responsibility but also realize that mistakes are inevitable. I do not need to let it stop me from managing my behaviors geared toward optimal health and wellness.

2. Inform _____ of my lapse and seek his/ her support.

3. Contact my support person to talk about it.

   • To figure out how it happened.

   • To figure out how it could be prevented next time, and what I will need to do differently.

Early Warning Signs

Early Warning Signs	Thoughts and Feelings	Coping Strategy

Triggers

Trigger	Thoughts and Feelings	Coping Strategy

High Risk Situations

Location	People	Circumstances	Coping Strategy

What do I get out of this behavior?

There are reasons for my behavior. Incentives exist or I wouldn't engage in it.

1. _____

2. _____

3. _____

4. _____

5. _____

6. _____

7. _____

I will take care of myself in these alternative ways (I know eating may seem like the best strategy in the short-term, but what really needs my attention for the best long-term results?):

1. _____

2. _____

3. _____

4. _____

5. _____

6. _____

7. _____

Motivation versus Commitment

Dieting and permanent weight loss requires a commitment to taking responsibility for one's health and wellness. For many individuals who begin a diet and set goals for adopting new skills, incorporating

healthier nutrition, and increasing activity, there is rarely an acknowledgement of the differences between motivation and commitment or a recognition for what responsibility-taking will look like as new habits are shaped and developed. Take a few minutes to identify what you believe to be your motivating factors for embarking on this journey. You might think in terms of each of your roles (i.e. mother, wife, teacher, brother, boss), the environments in which you spend your time (i.e. home, work, school), and the basic psychological needs universal to all human beings—autonomy, competence, and relatedness!

The factors motivating me to take this step include:

1. _____

2. _____

3. _____

4. _____

5. _____

Now, take a look at your list above and ask yourself if each factor is something that carries with it fleeting emotional weight or is something that makes you take stock 100% of the time. Is it always on your mind and at the forefront of everything you do? Is it an expression of your personal values or connected to compliance or conformity with others that doesn't feel congruent with your principles? Accordingly, assess whether these factors will result in a sense of confidence in your ability to navigate your life more effectively, in addition to generating a greater capacity to connect with others. If you identified any of the above as those that are constant drivers for healthy behavior, these would be better listed as those factors contributing to commitment-driven behavior. Commitment is what was described above as a pledge, an intrinsically oriented obligation, and total engagement. It is not short-term and swayed by our emotions like motivation is, but is instead, all-encompassing in nature. We do what we're committed to because we know it's in our best interest even if sometimes we "don't feel like it"; and because we are going to do it anyway, we find and create ways of making it fun. Now, identify those factors that will serve as committing forces for you as you move forward.

The factors that will commit me to achieve my goal of sustainable weight loss include:

1. _____

2. _____

3. _____

4. _____

5. _____

Developing a Plan for Hunger and Cravings

You have now shed some light on a few key factors that have contributed to your lack of success with previous dieting attempts. What many diets end up creating is deprivation and a severe lack of attunement to normal hunger signals. On a typical diet, one feels hungry and is trained to ignore it. Feelings of hunger are important as they provide signals that your body is in a particular state, necessary so that you can make a choice as to eat or wait, and opportunistic in that they allow you to become more aware of whether what you're experiencing is psychological or physiological.

Studies have shown that dieters, due to the restraint that most diets call for, tend to eat past the point of fullness when they eat slightly over what they have deemed appropriate. In essence, they adopt what is called the "dieter's mindset" and often say to themselves, "well, I already blew it, so I might as well eat a lot now before I get back to the diet." You can see how this mindset leads to a binge/restraint cycle and incorporates little flexibility for healthy management.

You may also be able to relate to the conundrum of not planning for incorporating the foods that you like. For example, if I'm going to eat a dessert, I want it to be rich, decadent, and dense. Anything less, and I'll likely be disappointed by it. Think back to the last time you said no to a food, telling yourself that it was off-limits. How much time did you spent obsessively thinking about it? I'm betting more than you were comfortable with. Now, think of a time when you told yourself that you couldn't have something you enjoyed, and you opted for something completely different "because it's healthy." I'm betting that later you went straight for the food you actually wanted, now having consumed two meals. I am not saying that all restraint is negative. Like managing your personal budget, you will have to implement discipline. Everything in moderation.

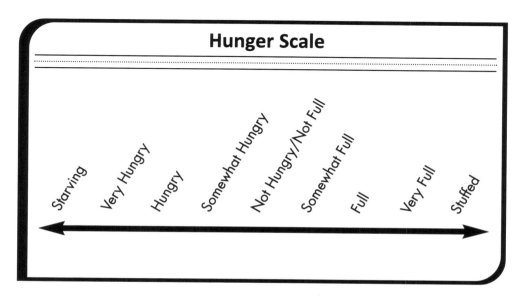

Hunger Scale

Starving — Very Hungry — Hungry — Somewhat Hungry — Not Hungry/Not Full — Somewhat Full — Full — Very Full — Stuffed

Hunger is normal. If it weren't, our bodies would not have developed the ability to tell you when your blood sugar has dropped and that it may be time to consider having a meal or snack. Hunger is largely physical—we experience feelings in our bodies indicating the condition. Cravings, on the other hand are connected to mood, to the situation, to our emotional states, and often manifest in a desire to eat something specific.

Developing a plan for managing hunger and cravings is crucial for success in losing weight as well as becoming more attuned to what your body and mind need.

Ask yourself the following questions to increase your personal awareness of hunger and its signals. Take your time. Notice over the course of the next few days as you decide to eat, why you're doing so, how you know it's time, or when you reach for food and notice that you're not hungry.

Do you know when you are hungry?

_____

_____

_____

_____

_____

How do you know when you are hungry? What happens inside your body to tell you?

_____

_____

_____

_____

_____

Do you eat when you are hungry?

_____

_____

_____

_____

_____

When you are hungry, what are your thoughts that guide your actions?

_____

_____

_____

_____

_____

Do you eat what you are hungry for, choosing from a wide variety of foods?

_____

_____

_____

_____

_____

Do you stop when you are full/satisfied?

_____

_____

_____

_____

_____

From here you can ask yourself what it is you really need. Often it is not food but instead something like sleep, connection, or comfort. Create a "toy box" of items that you can use to meet your needs rather than diving into food. Remember the three basic psychological needs of autonomy, competence, and relatedness/connection. Might your eating be related to one of these being threatened in some way?

Psychological Versus Physiological Hunger

It's helpful to rate your hunger when you have the urge to eat. You can use a scale such as the following to assess your hunger and to help you make a more mindful decision. People have communicated to me often that they do not know they are hungry until feeling headachy, lethargic, or perhaps a little shaky and feeling faint, and then it's too late. These are signals of hypoglycemia, and at this point hunger has become critical. In this situation, one feels a strong sense of urgency to eat whatever is put in front of them, and a wise decision is not as likely. When one does eat, the chances are high that more will be consumed than is necessary.

Rating your hunger can clue you into whether you are physically or psychologically hungry. You will use what you learned in the previous activity to assess the signs and symptoms your body is giving you.

Number the line above from 1 to 10.

1 will represent satisfaction and not being hungry at all.

10 would mean significant hunger.

5 would be somewhat neutral, for example, "I could eat, but I would be fine not eating also."

After numbering your scale, define at what numbers you would eat.

A client of mine described how if she rated herself anywhere between a 7-10, she would prepare a meal.

If she was anywhere between a 5-7, she might get a snack.

Lower than a 5, she would make a plan for eating later.

When we are speaking with each other, we assess the times when she would typically binge. That behavior would occur at night before going to bed. When she feels the urge to binge at this time now, she uses her scale to first assess physiologically if she needs to eat, and then psychologically assesses her current needs.

Asking the question, "If I'm not physically hungry right now, what is it that I'm really needing?" has made her pause and recognize that oftentimes she is anxious and feeling as if she shouldn't go to bed, that she should stay up and work. When she honors her fatigue and goes to bed instead of eating, she 1) takes care of herself in a healthy way; 2) proves to herself that she can listen to her body and not harm it; and 3) aligns herself with her goal of increased personal awareness.

As you practice more and become adept at reading your body's cues, a good rule of thumb for yourself might be that if you have to ask yourself if you're hungry, you probably aren't. We like to eat, and we can often justify eating even when we recognize we don't need it.

Identifying Barriers to Success

One of the oldest problem-solving interventions, but quite possibly one of the most effective, is brainstorming. A method of creatively assessing all the attributes attached to a central theme, brainstorming helps you to identify the parts of a single purpose. In this case, the theme we are using the brainstorming session for is *barriers to success*.

This activity is also very useful for identifying the contributing factors for events or behaviors that occur which are positive! We are going to call the activity *Completing a Fit*.

When you do this, you are asking yourself, "What's the fit of this situation?" and developing your list of everything you believe may have had an impact on your inability to reach your goals in the past. The idea is to look for areas that you can influence. Some things you list will not be in your control, for example, *there is no sidewalk around my house*, which you may have listed as a reason for not being able to exercise. Obviously, you cannot do anything about this, so while it may be valid, we look past it to the areas that you can impact. For example, *I was always hungry*. This is a common reason for dieting attempts to fail.

As you know, many diets are unrealistically restrictive and leave you feeling very low-energy and deprived. So this would be one area that you could develop new goals around and steps to take to ensure you are experiencing normal hunger. In this specific activity, you are identifying barriers to success in order to begin developing your plan for a more successful weight loss adventure. But the activity itself can be used any time you experience a set back or a *relapse*.

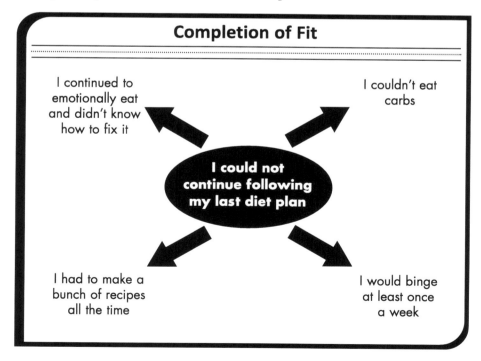

If you experienced a binge, this is a good place to start in working to recognize the antecedents to that behavior and tackle it head on. Using your challenges as opportunities to learn and grow is going to be in your best interest. So let's get started.

Think back to the last time you dieted. Assess from every environment, the contributing factors to the lack of success you experienced. Put yourself among friends, in social situations, at home, in restaurants, at school, with your family, at work, on vacation, at your doctor's office, in the gym, etc., and list every reason you can think of, even if it sounds far-fetched, that you did not succeed. You can do this in list format or like I have diagrammed below.

After you have exhausted all possibilities, circle two to four of them that you feel you can create new goals around to change their impact from negative to positive. You've learned a lot so far about physiology, food intake, thermogenesis, and blood sugar stability in tandem with the imperative psychological and behavioral components of successful dieting and weight maintenance.

Here's an example: "I couldn't eat carbs."

1. My new plan will contain carbohydrates within a healthy range.
2. I will give myself the flexibility to have some not-so-healthy types of carbs (like a peanut butter cub pre-workout) as well as healthier sources like fruits and vegetables.

Managing Emotions

Thoughts, feelings, and behaviors must be addressed for the purpose of increased awareness and solidification of commitment. Relapse is most often used in addiction literature, however, you can use this term to describe any action that puts you at risk of acting in a manner incongruent with your best interests.

Identify the thoughts you have used to justify actions that are not in line with your goals. Examples include:

I'll just have one.
I deserve this. I've worked so hard.
Nothing is working. I might as well...

1. _____
2. _____
3. _____
4. _____
5. _____

Consider the *event...thought....emotion....behavior* continuum. When an event occurs, you feel a certain way because of what your mind tells you. Often you relate a circumstance or a situation to something that happened in your past, and attach a meaning to it. Feelings are not inherently good or bad but are often perceived this way and lead to a desire to avoid or sustain them. You cannot control your feelings, but you can control your response. A few of the most common emotions that derail the best of intentions include sadness, anger, loneliness, fatigue, boredom and anxiety.

Looking at the thoughts you identified above, now identify your most common emotions that these thoughts lead to. Follow this up by assessing how you know you are feeling them. Signs are those indicators that can be seen on the outside (i.e. fidgeting, furrowed brow). Symptoms are signals occurring internally (i.e. tight chest, rapid heartbeat) and include your thoughts. Understanding your body's signals can clue you in to your emotions and aid in more automatic recognition. With practice, you will develop a more proactive, less impulsive response to them.

Emotions	Signs	Symptoms

Monitoring Cognitive Distortions

Negative thinking patterns often keep us locked into believing certain things about our abilities or the world around us, what we can or cannot do, and who we believe we should be. Practice recognizing the thoughts that you most often have that lead to justification of harmful behavior or acting in a way that is not congruent with your goals. Use the cognitive distortion list in Appendix E8 to assess how you might reframe your thoughts from a "just the facts" perspective. Examine the original thought and ask yourself, "Where is the evidence that this is true?"

Rethink Your Thoughts

Thought	Distortion	Reframe
I ate that cookie. Now the whole day is ruined.	Catastrophizing	It was one mistake. I still have all the good decisions made earlier!

Implementing Behavioral Flexibility

Studies demonstrate how behavioral flexibility plays a key role in mitigating the risks associated with relapse. One strategy for overcoming temptation and staying committed to your goals is to remind yourself of the reasons you have decided to change. Identify what might happen if you do not change (i.e. I will be diabetic) and how your life will be enhanced through commitment to your goals (i.e. I will be showing my kids how to be healthy for life).

If I veer off course and throw in the towel, the consequences may be:

1. _____

2. _____

3. _____

By sustaining commitment to my goals, I will achieve the following changes in my life:

1. _____

2. _____

3. _____

Reminding yourself of what ignites your desire can be thought of as *"playing it forward."*

Ask yourself, *"If I engage in this behavior* (i.e. eat outside of what I know will help me), *how will I feel emotionally and physically?"*

The above strategies are helpful for staying focused on the goals in front of you. However, taking the process a step further and identifying the rules that you may have in place that lead you toward behaviors that can undermine your success is important for creating a more flexible mindset.

Developing Problem-Solving Skills

It is human nature is to protect and deflect. Consider the fight-or-flight response. When danger is perceived, the body goes through a significant hormonal shift causing blood to be directed to the muscles and organs vital for keeping you alive. Forget about digesting your food if you're in a highly-stressful situation in which your body is anticipating an immediate threat! Most of the negative feelings that we perceive as threatening, however, are far from life-altering. Our knee-jerk reactions are often tied to distortions in thinking (Review the list of cognitive distortions in Appendix E8) and can challenge our ability to problem-solve effectively. Consider using the cognitive distortion list if you find yourself getting stuck during your problem-solving session.

RADAR

Skill: Recognize and Assess

Definition: Identifying that a problem exists or recognition of discomfort (or an emotion); approaching it as an opportunity, with curiosity, and a willingness to devote some attention, time and energy toward it.

Example: You're dieting and you're leaving for vacation in a week. You've acknowledged that you're nervous about feeling out of control around the food, as much of it you won't be cooking, and you don't want to come back ten pounds heavier like last time. You decide that you have enough time to anticipate and plan ahead and you determine that while the situation won't be your normal routine, it doesn't mean it will be "bad" or "wrong."

Skill: Deepen and Accept

Definition: Gather information to clearly understand the problem and the reasons behind your emotional response. Assess how the situation is different than you would like it to be in light of your goals. Objectively prioritize your needs in order of importance. Identify the situation with a "just the facts" approach to remove the unrealistic "out of control" feeling you may be experiencing. Deepen the level of compassion you have for yourself through monitoring the self-talk you are engaging in and create a container for your experience.

Example: Perhaps the situation is causing stress due to your perception of it. Maybe you think that not sticking to your typical eating schedule or that not having a gym to work out in is going to make you gain weight. These differences are valid, however, the assumption that you'll gain weight is not. To assess the objectivity of your thoughts, ask yourself, "Where is the evidence that this is true?" Assess how you might continue exercising but in a different manner while you're gone and make a plan for how you will modify your food intake in light of the decrease in activity and differences in food choices. Finally, recognize that you are reacting this way because your goal is important to you. You are your advocate!

Skill: Reflect and Respond

Definition: Ask yourself what has worked well in the past in similar situations and how you can apply the same tactics. Generate alternative solutions and don't limit yourself. Play each possible action forward and ask yourself, "If I do this, how will I feel afterward?" Respond unemotionally, with your goals at the forefront of your mind. Reach out and gather additional resources, be those people or previous experiences that you can draw on for strength, or even images that enable you to feel a sense of calm and confidence in what is ahead. They do not have to be related to the challenge at hand. Bringing to mind your child's smile or the way your partner brushed your hair away from your face gently before he kissed you goodnight can bring a sense of peace that you may need to think more clearly.

Example: You could call ahead to book a hotel that has a fitness room, get on the internet and look up the restaurants that surround the area you're staying in, and make a list of foods you could pack to take with you that could help you to stay on track in between your "out" meals. If you know, perhaps, that you'll be going to Cheesecake Factory and that you'll not want to try to resist the cheesecake (C'mon, some things you just DO NOT give up!), consider having the dessert itself for dinner and having a small house salad beforehand as your "meal." Think outside the box. Reflect on whether the choices you are considering are in your best interest and are congruent with your best self.

Skill: Revise

Definition: After implementing your strategy, it's time to examine its effectiveness. How well did your decision solve the problem? What methods did you use to get into an effective mindset? Could you change it in any way? What specifically went well, and how might you develop your strategy further?

Example: You encountered moments during your trip that were not necessarily "easy" to navigate, but you made sure to pause before making any knee-jerk, impulsive reactions. You did end up going to Cheesecake Factory, and while you made the choice to have dinner *and* dessert and felt a bit too full afterward, you didn't follow that meal up with another day of free eating. Thinking about how you could have approached that meal differently, you decide that next time you'll ask for some support from your partner before you go.

Anticipating and Planning Ahead

Whenever you start down the path of changing habits and creating new behaviors, you can expect "relapse." Many of our behaviors are automatic due to their repeated use. To change requires intentional, deliberate, conscious action. Anticipating what might cause you some difficulty as you progress allows you to identify how you could respond proactively and avoid a setback. For example, the dieter may attend a party and see an array of her old favorite snack foods and feel tempted to stray from her nutrition structure. Use previous experiences to identify your triggers. Otherwise known as threats, triggers may include people, places, foods, smells, etc.

Trigger 1: _____

Trigger 2: _____

Trigger 3: _____

Trigger 4: _____

Trigger 5: _____

Skills Transfer

As you begin considering weight loss and dieting, it is not unusual to feel overwhelmed with the tasks ahead. Especially if you are someone who has engaged in numerous attempts at dieting only to see your weight come back, I would expect that you anticipate failure much more so than success! However, other programs you've tried did not likely include a focus on education within both the physiological and psychological realms. Additionally, most individuals have not considered the skills associated with dieting. Going into weight loss with the assumption that *I just have to burn more than I eat* will not net you permanent success. Many of you already know this—it is one reason why you are reading this book and digging into these activities.

I am going to assume that each of you has accomplished something big in your life. You set a goal, you took steps toward that goal, and at some point, no matter how long it took you, the goal was achieved. These goals could include having and raising children, finding your spouse, earning a degree, learning a new song on the guitar, or anything meaningful to you.

Perhaps you had to take a different route somewhere in the middle of your course. Maybe you veered off your anticipated path a few times and had to solicit some help. Nonetheless, you made it. Throughout your journey you implemented various skills and you learned some new ones along the way. Identifying these skills is crucial now to adopting a sound mindset and strategy for weight loss!

You can apply what you already possess to successfully navigate the challenges ahead. Take some time now to jot down the skills or traits you possess or have applied toward previous achievements. They may include specific behaviors such as time blocking, preparing meals ahead of time, and shutting off the phone to eliminate distractions while studying; or they can be traits such as patience, determination, or passion. Don't forget to think about what you do in your day to day work—an engineer I worked with found great success when he approached his weight loss goal the same way he does job responsibilities! Go!

1. _____

2. _____

3. _____

4. _____

5. _____

6. _____

7. _____

8. _____

Now, reread each item above and list how you can apply it in this context. The most successful dieters I have worked with have done this activity a few times throughout their work with me. As they evolve and learn more about what behaviors fit best with them, and as they try on new hats and discover the various impacts of different tools, they sink into behaviors that fit who they are rather than trying to shove themselves into someone else's box.

Using Setbacks to Improve Future Behavior

Over the next two weeks as you are meeting people, talking to them, going to the gym, shopping at the store, watching television, etc., assess the personalities, characteristics, and lifestyles of others. What do they do, how do they act, and how do they carry themselves?

We often admire in others what is similar in our own lives, or, importantly, what we would appreciate having in our lives. With practice, you can embody the behaviors you admire in others. Sometimes it takes acting "as if."

If you said that your best friend is creative, break this down. Get specific. You do not have to be creative in home design like he is; perhaps you enjoy cooking and want to take this to a new level. What is one thing you can do to ramp up your creativity in the kitchen?

Identify three things that you would like to emulate, and for each of those three things, identify two ways in which you could learn more about how to begin becoming this person.

1. _____

   a. _____

   b. _____

2. _____

   a. _____

   b. _____

3. _____

   a. _____

   b. _____

Exercise

How might each of the cognitive distortions undermine your confidence in meeting the challenges associated with your health goals? Identify the thoughts you have that fit each distortion as they relate to exercise. If you easily counteract them at this point, what do you say to yourself?

Cognitive Distortions

All-or-nothing thinking (splitting)—Thinking of things in absolute terms, like "always", "every", "never", and "there is no alternative." Few aspects of human behavior are so absolute. All-or-nothing-thinking can contribute to depression.

Overgeneralization—Taking isolated cases and using them to make sweeping generalizations.

Mental filter—Focusing almost exclusively on certain, usually negative or upsetting, aspects of an event while ignoring other positive aspects. For example, focusing on a tiny imperfection in a piece of otherwise useful clothing.

Disqualifying the positive—Continually reemphasizing or "shooting down" positive experiences for arbitrary, ad hoc reasons.

Jumping to conclusions—Drawing conclusions (usually negative) from little (if any) evidence. Two specific subtypes are also identified:

Mind reading—Assuming special knowledge of the intentions or thoughts of others.

Fortune telling—Exaggerating how things will turn out before they happen.

Magnification and **minimization**—Distorting aspects of a memory or situation through magnifying or minimizing them such that they no longer correspond to objective reality. This is common enough in the normal population to popularize idioms such as "make a mountain out of a molehill." In depressed clients, often the positive characteristics of *other people* are exaggerated and negative characteristics are understated. There is one subtype of magnification:

Catastrophizing—Focusing on the worst possible outcome, however unlikely, or thinking that a situation is unbearable or impossible when it is really just uncomfortable.

Emotional reasoning—Making decisions and arguments based on intuitions or personal *feeling* rather than an objective rationale and evidence.

Should statements—Patterns of thought which imply the way things "should" or "ought to be" rather than the actual situation the patient is faced with or having rigid rules which one believes will "always apply" no matter what the circumstances are.

Labeling and mislabeling—Explaining behaviors or events, merely by naming them; related to overgeneralization. Rather than describing the specific behavior, one assigns a label to someone of him- or herself that implies absolute and unalterable terms. Mislabeling involves describing an event with language that is highly colored and emotionally loaded.

Personalization—Attribution of personal responsibility (or causal role) for events over which one has no control. This pattern is also applied to others in the attribution of blame.

Rethink Your Thoughts

Thought	Distortion	Reframe
I'm too tired to exercise.	Emotional Reasoning	Exercise will help to energize me.

Develop Commitment
through a Strong Support System

Assess what you would like to tell others you are doing. Clearly stating your goals makes them more prominent and puts you in a position of power.

Next, consider the reactions you might receive from others. Identify the questions and comments you may hear from friends, family, and even those who witness the changes in your body and attitude and ask what you are doing. Then identify how you might respond. It's not uncommon for those who lose weight to receive comments that are quite surprising and sometimes less than flattering.

Comments I might receive from others (consider praise, questions, criticisms, etc.):

1. _____

My response:

2. _____

My response:

3. _____

My Response:

4. _____

My Response:

5. _____

My Response:

6. _____

My Response:

Finally, complete a support assessment. Who and what can you draw on when you need assistance, a pick-me-up, a swift-kick, or an "atta boy"? Don't stop there though. List specifically what you will ask for from these people. Put yourself in their shoes and consider the energy that they might have to exert in helping you. Last but not least, request their help!

Support People

Person: _____

Contact Details: _____

What I will ask for: _____

How I will ask: _____

How I might repay them: _____

Person: _____

Contact Details: _____

What I will ask for: _____

How I will ask: _____

How I might repay them: _____

BIBLIOGRAPHY

Abbasi, F., et al. (2000). High carbohydrate diets, triglyceride rich lipoproteins, and coronary heart disease risk. *American Journal of Cardiology, 85*, 45-48.

Abbott, D.W., et al. (1998). Onset of binge eating and dieting in overweight women: Implications for etiology, associated features and treatment. *Journal of Psychosomatic Research, 44*(¾), 367–374.

Acheson, K.J., et al. (1984). Nutritional influences on lipogenesis and thermogenesis after a carbohydrate meal. *American Journal of Physiology, 246*, E62-E70.

Agus, M.S.D., et al. (2000). Dietary composition and physiologic adaptations to energy restriction. *American Journal of Clinical Nutrition, 71*, 901-907.

Alonso-Tapia, J., Huertas, J.A., & Ruiz, M.A. (2010). On the nature of motivational orientations: Implications of assessed goals and gender differences for motivational goal theory. *The Spanish Journal of Psychology, 13*(1), 232-243.

Anderson-Fye, E.P., & Becker, A.E. (2004). Sociocultural aspects of eating disorders. In Thompson, K.J. (Ed.), *Handbook of eating disorders and obesity* (pp. 565-589). Hoboken, NJ: John Wiley & Sons.

Appelhans, B.M., Whited, M.C., Schneider, K.L., Oleski, J., & Pagoto, S.L. (2011). Response style and vulnerability to anger-induced eating in obese adults. *Eating Behavior, 12*(1), 9-14. doi:10.1016/j.eatbeh.2010.08.009

Ascherio, A., & Willet, W.C. (1997). Health effects of transfatty acids. *American Journal of Clinical Nutrition, 66*, 1006S-1010S.

Atkins, R.C. (2002). *Dr. Atkins' new diet revolution.* New York, NY: Avon.

Baba, N.H., et al. (1999). High protein versus high carbohydrate hypoenergetic diet for the treatment of obese hyperinsulinemic subjects. *International Journal of Obesity, 11*, 1202-1206.

Bartholomew, K.J., Ntoumanis, N., Ryan, R.M., & Thogersen-Ntoumani, C. (2011). Psychological need thwarting in the sport context: Assessing the darker side of athletic experience. *Journal of Sport & Exercise Psychology, 33*, 75-102.

Baumeister, R.F. (2002a). Ego depletion and self-control failure: An energy model of self's executive function. *Self and Identity, 2*(April), 129-136.

Baumeister, R.F. (2002b). Yielding to temptation: Self control failure, impulsive purchasing, and consumer behavior. *Journal of Consumer Research, 28*(March), 670-676.

Befort, C.A., Stewart, E.E., Smith, B.K., Gibson, C.A., Sullivan, D.K., & Donnelly, J.E. (2008). Weight maintenance, behaviors and barriers among previous participants of a university-based weight control program. *International Journal of Obesity, 32*, 519-526. doi:10.1038/sj.ijo.0803769

Bell, C.G., Walley, A.J., & Froguel, P. (2005). The genetics of human obesity. *Nature Reviews/ Genetics 6*, 221.

Bennett, J., Greene, G., & Schwartz-Barcott, D. (2013). Perceptions of emotional eating behavior: A qualitative study of college students. *Appetite, 60*(1), 187-192.

Benoit, S.C., Davis, J.E., & Davidson, T.L. (2010). Learned and cognitive controls of food intake. *Brain Research, 1350*, 71-76.

Berthoud, H-R. (2004). Mind versus metabolism in the control of food intake and energy balance. *Physiology & Behavior, 81,* 781– 793.

Bisogni, C.A., Connors, M., Devine, C.M., & Sobal, J. (2002). Who we are and how we eat: A qualitative study of identities in food choice. *Journal of Nutrition Education and Behavior, 34,* 128-139.

Blocher, McCabe, E., Kavia, M.C., & Marcus, M.D. (2004). Dialectical behavior therapy for eating disorders. In K.J. Thompson (Ed.), *Handbook of eating disorders and obesity* (pp. 232-244). Hoboken, NJ: John Wiley & Sons.

Boeije, H. (2010). *Analysis in qualitative research.* Los Angeles, CA: Sage Publications.

Boggiano, M.M., Dorsey, J.R., Thomas, J.M., & Murdaugh, D.L. (2009). The Pavlovian power of palatable food: Lessons for weight-loss adherence from a new rodent model of cue-induced overeating. *International Journal of Obesity (London), 33*(6), 693-701.

Bolger, N., Davis, A., & Rafaeili, E. (2003). Diary methods: Capturing life as it is lived. *Annual Review of Psychology, 54,* 579-616.

Bongaard, B. (2008, July/August). Mind over cupcake [Diet and Nutrition]. *Explore, 4*(4), 267-272.

Brand-Miller, J.C. et al. (2002). Glycemic index and obesity. *American Journal of Clinical Nutrition, 76,* 281S-285S.

Brand-Miller, J., et al. (2003). *The New Glucose Revolution.* Marlowe and Company: New York, NY.

Bravata, D.M., Sanders, Huang, et al. (2003). Efficacy and safety of low-carbohydrate diets: A systematic review. *Journal of the American Medical Association, 289*(14):1837-1850.

Bray, G.A. (1969). Effect of caloric restrictions on energy expenditure in obese patients. *Lancet, 2,* 397-398.

Bray, G.A. (2003). Low-carbohydrate diets and realities of weight loss. *Journal of the American Medical Association, 289*(14), 1853-1855.

Bray, G.A., & Champagne, C.M. (2005). Beyond energy balance: There is more to obesity than kilocalories. *Journal of the American Dietetic Association, 105,* S17-S23.

Brody, T. (1999). *Nutritional biochemistry,* (5th ed.). San Diego, CA: Academic Press.

Brownell, K.D., Greenwood, Stellar, & Shrager (1986). The effects of repeated cycles of weight loss and regain in rats. *Physiology Behavior, 38,* 459-464.

Buckroyd, J., Rother, S., & Stott, D. (2006). Weight loss as a primary objective of therapeutic groups for obese women: Two preliminary studies. *British Journal of Guidance & Counselling, 34*(2), 245-265. doi:10.1080/03069880600583303

Burnard, P. (1991). A method of analyzing interview transcripts in qualitative research. *Nurse Education Today, 11*, 461-466.

Burton, P., Smit, H.J., & Lightowler, H.J. (2007). The influence of restrained and external eating patterns on overeating. *Appetite, 49*, 191-197.

Butryn, M.L., Thomas, J.G., & Lowe, M.R. (2009). Reductions in internal disinhibition during weight loss predict better weight loss maintenance. *Obesity, 17*, 1101-1103. doi: 10.1038/oby.2008.646

Byrne, S., Cooper, Z., & Fairburn, C. (2003). Weight maintenance and relapse in obesity: A qualitative study. *International Journal of Obesity, 27*, 955-962.

Campfield, L., Smith, & Burn (1998). Strategies and potential molecular targets for obesity treatment. *Science, 280*, 1383-1387.

Campos, P. (2005, October 7). The obesity myth: The 'war on fat' is a witch hunt masquerading as a public health initiative. *Spiked-online.com*. Retrieved from Retrieved from http://www.spiked-online.com/articles/0000000CADA2.htm

Carlola, R., Harley, & Noback (1990). *Human Anatomy and Physiology*. New York, NY: McGraw-Hill.

Chinachoti, P. (1995). Carbohydrates: Functionality in foods. *American Journal of Clinical Nutrition, 61*, 922S-929S.

Ciarrochi, J., Hynes, K., & Crittenden, N. (2005). Can men do better if they try harder: Sex and motivational effects on emotional awareness. *Cognition and Emotion, 19*(1), 133-141. doi: 10.1080/02699930441000102

Clark, L.T., Ferdinand, & Ferdinand (2003). *Contemporary management of the metabolic syndrome*. New York, NY: McMahon Publishing Group.

Costanzo, P.R., Musante, G.J., Friedman, K.E., Kern, L.S., & Tomlinson, K. (1999). The gender specificity of emotional, situational, and behavioral indicators of binge eating in a diet-seeking obese population. *International Journal of Eating Disorders, 26*, 205-210.

Crapo, P.A. (1985). Simple versus complex carbohydrate use in the diabetic diet. *Annual Review of Nutrition, 5*, 95-114.

Creswell, J.W. (2009).Writing strategies and ethical considerations. In Creswell, J.W. (Ed.), *Research design: Qualitative, quantitative, and mixed methods approaches* (pp. 75-94). Thousand Oaks, CA: Sage Publications, Inc.

Daly, M.E., et al. (1997). Dietary carbohydrate and insulin sensitivity: A review of the evidence and clinical implications. *American Journal of Clinical Nutrition, 66*, 1072-1085.

Davis, C. (2001, February). Addiction and the eating disorders. *Psychiatric Times, (18)*2. Retrieved from http://www.psychiatrictimes.com/display/article/10168/54311

Depres, J.P., et al. (1996). Hyperinsulinemia as an independent risk factor for ischemic heart disease. *New England Journal of Medicine, 334,* 952-957.

De Ridder, D., Kuijer, R., & Ouwehand, C. (2007). Does confrontation with potential goal failure promote self-regulation? Examining the role of distress in the pursuit of weight goals. *Psychology and Health, 22*(6), 677-698. doi:10.1080/14768320601020238

de Souza, P., & Ciclitira, K.E. (2005). Men and dieting: A qualitative analysis. *Journal of Health Psychology, 10,* 793-804.

De Zwaan, M., Roerig, J.L., & Mitchell, J.E. (2004). Pharmacological treatment of anorexia nervosa, bulimia nervosa, and binge eating disorder. In K.J. Thompson (Ed.), *Handbook of eating disorders and obesity* (pp. 186-217). Hoboken, NJ: John Wiley & Sons.

Diamond, D.M., Campbell, A.M., Park, C.R., Halonen, J., & Zoladz, P.R. (2007). The temporal dynamics model of emotional memory processing: A synthesis of the neurobiological basis of stress-induced amnesia, flashbulb and traumatic memories, and the Yerkes-Dodson law. *Neural Plasticity,* (60803).

Dune, L.J. (1990). *Nutrition almanac,* (3rd ed.). New York, NY: McGraw-Hill.

Draper, A., & Swift, J.A. (2010). Qualitative research in nutrition and dietetics: Data collection issues. *Journal of Human Nutrition and Dietetics, 24,* 3-12.

Eades, M.R., & Eades (1996). *Protein power.* New York, NY: Bantam Books.

Eaton, R., & Bradley, G. (2008). The role of gender and negative affectivity in stressor appraisal and coping selection. *International Journal of Stress Management, 15*(1), 94-115.

Elfhag, K. & Rossner, S. (2005). Who succeeds in maintaining weight loss? A conceptual review of factors associated with weight loss maintenance and weight regain. *Obesity Reviews, 6,* 67-85.

Elo, S., & Kyngas, H. (2007). The qualitative content analysis process. *Journal of Advanced Nursing, 62*(1), 107-115.

Ely, D.L. (1997). Overview of dietary sodium effects on and interactions with cardiovascular and neuroendocrine functions. *American Journal of Clinical Nutrition, 65,* 594S-605S.

Erikson, R.H., & Kim, Y.S. (1990). Digestion and absorption of dietary protein. *Annual Review of Medicine, 41,* 133-139.

Fabes, R.A., & Eisenberg, N. (1997). Regulatory control and adults' stress-related responses to daily life events. *Journal of Personality and Social Psychology, 73*(5), 1107-1117.

Felig, P., et al. (1970). Amino acid metabolism in the regulation of gluconeogenesis in man. *American Journal of Clinical Nutrition, 23,* 986-992.

Felig, P., Baxter, J.D., & Frohman, L.A. (1995). *Endocrinology and metabolism,* (3rd ed.). New York, NY: McGraw-Hill.

Figlewicz, D.P., et al. (1996). Endocrine regulation of food intake and body weight. *Journal of Laboratory and Clinical Medicine, 127,* 328-332.

Fisler, J.S., et al. (1982). Nitrogen economy during very low calorie reducing diets. *American Journal of Clinical Nutrition, 35,* 471-486.

Flegal, K.M., Carroll, M.D., Ogden, C.L., & Curtin, L.R. (2010). Prevalence and trends in obesity among U.S. adults, 1999-2008. *Journal of the American Medical Association, 303*(3), 235-241.

Flegal, K.M., Graubard, B.I., Williamson, D.F., & Gail, M.H. (2005). Excess deaths associated with underweight, overweight, and obesity. *Journal of the American Medical Association, 293,* 15, 1861-1868.

Fletcher, B., Hanson, J., Page, N., & Pine, K. (2011). FIT- Do something different: A new behavioral program for sustained weight loss. *Swiss Journal of Psychology, 70*(1), 25-34. doi:10.1024/1421-0185/a000035

Ford, E.S., & Liu, S. (2001). Glycemic index and serum high-density-lipoprotein cholesterol concentration among US adults. *Archives of Internal Medicine, 161,* 572-578.

Fordslund, A.H., et al. (1999). Effect of protein intake and physical activity on twenty-four hour pattern and rate of micronutrient utilization. *American Physiology Society,* E964-E976.

Foster-Powell, K., Brand-Miller, J.C., & Holt, S.H.A. (2002). International table of glycemic index and glycemic load values. *American Journal of Clinical Nutrition, 76,* 5-56.

Framson, C., Kristal, A.R., Schenk, J.M., Littman, A.J., Zeliadt, S., & Benitez, D. (2009). Development and validation of the mindful eating questionnaire. *Journal of the American Dietetic Association, 109,* 1439-1444. doi:10.1016/j.jada.2009.05.006

Franko, D.L., Wonderlich, S.A., Little, D., & Herzog, D.B. (2004). Diagnosis and classification of eating disorders. In Thompson, K.J. (Ed.), *Handbook of eating disorders and obesity* (pp. 58-80). Hoboken, NJ: John Wiley & Sons.

Fraser, G.E., Sabate, J., Beeson, W.L., & Strahan, T.M. (1992). A possible protective effect of nutrition consumption on risk of coronary heart disease—The Adventist Health Study. *Archives of Internal Medicine, 152,* 1416-1424.

Freeman, M., deMarrais, K., Preissle, J., Roulston, K., & St. Pierre, E.A. (2007). Standards of evidence in qualitative research: An incitement to discourse. *Educational Researcher, 36*(1), 25-32. doi:10.3102/0013189X06298009

Friedman, H.I., & Nylund, B. (1980). Intestinal fat digestion, absorption, and transport. *American Journal of Clinical Nutrition, 33,* 1108-1139.

Friedman, M.A., & Brownell, K.D. (1995). Psychological correlates of obesity: Moving to the next research generation. *Psychological Bulletin, 117*(1), 3-20.

Frost, G., & Dornhorst, A. (2000). The relevance of the glycemic index to our understanding of dietary carbohydrates. *Diabetic Medicine, 17*, 336-345.

Fujita, K. (2011). On conceptualizing self-control as more than the effortful inhibition of impulses. *Personality and Social Psychology Review, 15*, 352-366. doi: 10.1177/1088868311411165

Fushiki, T., et al. (1989). Changes in glucose transporters in muscle in response to glucose. *American Journal of Physiology, 256*, E580-E587.

Gladis, M.M., Wadden, T.A., Vogt, R., Foster, G., Kuehnel, R.H., & Bartlett, S.J. (1998). Behavioral treatment of obese binge eaters: Do they need different care? *Journal of Psychosomatic Research, 44*(¾), 375–384.

Golay, A., et al. (1996). Weight loss with low or high carbohydrate diet? *International Journal of Obesity and Related Metabolic Disorders, 20*, 1067-1072.

Gold, M.S., Frost-Pineda, K., & Jacobs, W.S. (2003, February). Overeating, binge eating, and eating disorders as addictions. *Psychiatric Annals, (33)*2, 117-123. Retrieved from http://proquest.umi.com.proxy1.ncu.edu/pqdweb?did=290008861&sid=1&Fmt=4&clientld=52110&RQT=309&VName=PQD

Goldman, L., & Bennett, J.C. (2000). *Cecil textbook of medicine,* (21st ed.). Philadelphia, PA: Saunders.

Gorin, A.A., Powers, T.A., Koestner, R., Wing, R.R., & Raynor, H.A. (2013). Autonomy

support, self-regulation, and weight loss. *Health Psychology*, online, 1-8. doi:10.1037/a0032586

Gottfried, S.S. (1993). *Biology today.* St. Louis, MO: Mosby.

Groff, J.L., & Gropper, S.S. (2000). *Advanced nutrition and human metabolism.* Stamford, CT: Wadsworth Thomson Learning.

Gross, L.S., Ford, E.S., & Liu, S. (2004). Increased consumption of refined carbohydrates and the epidemic of type 2 diabetes in the United States: An ecologic assessment. *American Journal of Clinical Nutrition, 79*, 774-779.

Hagger, M.S., Chatzisarantis, N.L.D., & Harris, J. (2006). From psychological needs satisfaction to intentional behavior: Testing motivational sequences in two behavioral contexts. *Personality and Social Psychology Bulletin, 32*, 131-148.

Hardcastle, S., & Hagger, M.S. (2011). "You can't do it on your own": Experiences of a motivational interviewing intervention on physical activity and dietary behavior. *Psychology of Sport and Exercise, 12*, 314-323.

Hatahet, M.A., & Dhurandhar, N.V. (2004). Assessment of medical status and physical factors. In K.J. Thompson (Ed.), *Handbook of eating disorders and obesity* (pp. 372-392). Hoboken, NJ: John Wiley & Sons.

Head, S. (2002). Binge eating in obesity: Treatment and weight management issues. *Healthy Weight Journal, 16*(3), 24-26.

Heatherton, T.F., & Baumeister, R.F. (1991). Binge eating as escape from self-awareness. *Psychological Bulletin, 110,* 86-108.

Heatherton, T.F., Herman, C.P., & Polivy, J. (1991). Effects of physical threat and ego threat on eating. *Journal of Personality and Social Psychology, 60,* 138-143.

Henderson, K.E., & Brownell, K.D. (2004). The toxic environment and obesity: Contribution and cure. In K.J. Thompson (Ed.), *Handbook of eating disorders and obesity* (pp. 339-348). Hoboken, NJ: John Wiley & Sons.

Henwood, K.L., & Pidgeon, N.F. (1992). Qualitative research and psychological theorizing. *British Journal of Psychology, 83,* 97-111.

Hindle, L., & Carpenter, C. (2011). An exploration of the experiences and perceptions of people who have maintained weight loss. *Journal of Human Nutrition and Dietetics, 24,* 342-350.

Hohlstein, L.A., Smith, G.T., & Atlas, J.G. (1998). An application of expectancy theory to eating disorders: Development and validation of measures of eating and dieting expectancies. *Psychological Assessments, 10,* 49-58.

Holloszy, J., & Kohrt, W. (1996). Regulation of carbohydrate and fat metabolism during and after exercise. *Annual Review of Nutrition, 16,* 121-138.

Holman, R.T. (1988). George O. Burr and the discovery of essential fatty acids. *Journal of Nutrition, 118,* 535-540.

Hormone regulates fondness for food. (2007, August 11). *ScienceDaily.* Retrieved from http://www.sciencedaily.com/releases/2007/08/070809172258.htm

Hu, F.B., Willett, W.C., Li, T., et al. (2004). Adiposity as compared with physical activity in predicting mortality among women. *New England Journal of Medicine, 351,* 2694-2703.

Hudgins, L., et al. (2000). Relationship between carbohydrate induced hypertriglyceridemia and fatty acid synthesis in lean and obese subjects. *Journal of Lipid Research, 41,* 595-604.

Ingledew, D., & Markland, D. (2009). Three levels of motivation. *Applied Psychology, 3,* 336-355.

Jacobson, M.F., & Hurley, J. (2002). *Restaurant confidential.* New York, NY: Workman Publishing.

Jenkins, D.J., Kendall, C.W, Marchie, A., & Augustin, L.S. (2004). Too much sugar, too much carbohydrate, or just too much? *American Journal of Clinical Nutrition, 79,* 711-712.

Jones, P. (2006, February 2). Big, fat lie? Professor: 'Obesity epidemic' is a myth. *Knight Ridder Tribune Business News* [Wire feed], p. 1. Retrieved from http://proquest.umi.com.proxy1.ncu.edu/pqdweb?did=980676331&sid=5&Fmt=3&clientld=52110&RQT=309&VName=PQD

Karasu, S.R. (2012). Of mind and matter: Psychological dimensions in obesity. *American Journal of Psychotherapy, 66*(2), 111-128.

Kelly, J.F., & Hoeppner, B.B. (2013). Does Alcoholics Anonymous work differently for men and women? A moderated multiple-mediation analysis in a large clinical sample. *Drug and Alcohol Dependence, 130,* 186-193. doi:10.1016/j.drugalcdep.2012.11.005

Kelly, M.M., Tyrka, A.R., Anderson, G.M., Price, L.H., Carpenter, L.L. (2007). Sex differences in emotional and physiological responses to the Trier Social Stress Test. *Journal of Behavior Therapy and Experimental Psychiatry, 39,* 87-98.

Kemp, E., Bui, M., & Grier, S. (2011). Eating their feelings: Examining emotional eating in at-risk groups in the United States. *Journal of Consumer Policy, 34,* 211-229. doi:10.1007/s10603-010-0149-y

Khong, B.S.L. (2011). Mindfulness: A way of cultivating deep respect for emotions. *Mindfulness, 2,* 27-32. doi:10.1007/s12671-010-0039-9

Kristeller, J.L., & Hallett, C.B. (1999). An exploratory study of a meditation-based intervention for binge eating disorder. *Journal of Health Psychology, 4*(3), 357-363.

Kristeller, J.L., & Wolever, R.Q. (2010). Mindfulness-based eating awareness training for treating binge eating disorder: The conceptual foundation. *Eating Disorders, 19*(1), 49-61. doi:10.1080/106 40266.2011.533605

Kristeller, J.L., Baer, R.A., & Wolever, R.Q. (2006). Mindfulness-based approaches to eating disorders. In Baer, R. (Ed.). *Mindfulness and acceptance-based interventions: Conceptualization, application, and empirical support.* San Diego, CA: Elsevier.

Lally, P., Wardle, J., & Gardner, B. (2011). Experiences of habit formation: A qualitative study. *Psychology, Health & Medicine, 16*(4), 484-489. doi:10.1080/13548506.2011.555774

Larsen, J.K., van Strien, T., Eisinga, R., & Engels, R.C.M.E. (2006). Gender differences in the association between alexithymia and emotional eating in obese individuals. *Journal of Psychosomatic Research, 60,* 237-243.

Leaf, A., & Weber, P.C. (1988). Cardiovascular effects of n-3 fatty acids. *New England Journal of Medicine, 318,* 549-557.

Leeds, A.R. (2002). Glycemic index and heart disease. *American Journal of Clinical Nutrition, 76,* 286S-289S.

Leibel, R.L., Rosenbaum, M., & Hirsch, J. (1995). Changes in energy expenditure resulting from altered body weight. *New England Journal of Medicine, 332,* 621-628.

Leibowitz, S.F. (1992). Neurochemical-neuroendocrine systems in the brain controlling macronutrient intake and metabolism. *Trends in Neuroscience, 15,* 491-497.

Lillis, J., Hayes, S.C., Bunting, K., & Masuda, A. (2009). Teaching acceptance and mindfulness to improve the lives of the obese: A preliminary test of a theoretical model. *Annals of Behavioral Medicine: A Publication of the Society of Behavioral Medicine, 37,* 58-69. doi: 10.1007/s12160-009-9083x. Retrieved September 9, 2010, from the PsycARTICLES database.

Lindvall, K., Larsson, C., Weinehall, L., & Emmelin, M. (2010). Weight maintenance as a tight rope walk- a grounded theory study. *BMC Public Health, 10*(51), 1-11.

Liu, Simmin, W.C., Willett, J.E., Manson, et al. (2003). Relation between changes in intakes in dietary fiber and grain products and changes in weight and development of obesity among middle aged women. *American Journal of Clinical Nutrition, 78*, 920-927.

Lock, J. (2004). Family approaches for anorexia nervosa and bulimia nervosa. In K.J. Thompson (Ed.), *Handbook of eating disorders and obesity* (pp. 218-231). Hoboken, NJ: John Wiley & Sons.

Logue, A. (1991). *The psychology of eating and drinking: An introduction* (2nd ed.). New York, NY: W H Freeman/Times Books/ Henry Holt & Co. Retrieved from PsycINFO database.

Lutz, A., Slagter, H.A., Dunne, J.D., & Davidson, R.J. (2008). Attention regulation and monitoring in meditation. *Trends in Cognitive Sciences, 12*(4), 163-169.

Mann, T., Tomiyama, A., Westling, E., Lew, A., Samuels, B., & Chatman, J. (2007). Medicare's search for effective obesity treatments: Diets are not the answer. *American Psychologist, 62*(3), 220-233. doi:10.1037/0003-066X.62.3.220

Mardiah, B.A., Hazizi, A.S., Nasir, M.T.M., & Jan, J.M.H. (2012). Gender differences in the attitude and strategy towards weight control among government employees in Penang, Malaysia. *Iranian Journal of Public Health, 41*(1), 28-36.

McArdle, W.D., Katch, F.I., & Katch, V.L. (1991). *Exercise Physiology: Energy, Nutrition, and Human Performance,* Third ed. Lea and Febiger: Malvern, PA.

McCabe, M.P. & Ricciardelli, L.A. (2004). Weight and shape concerns of boys and men. In Thompson, K.J. (Ed.), *Handbook of eating disorders and obesity* (pp. 606-634). Hoboken, NJ: John Wiley & Sons.

McCall, T. (March/April 2005). Relax and unload. *Yoga Journal, 14*.

McGrath, J., & Johnson, B. (2003). Methodology makes meaning: How both qualitative and quantitative paradigms shape evidence and its interpretation. Camic, P., Rhodes, J., & Yardley, L. (Eds.), *Qualitative research in psychology: Expanding perspectives in methodology and design* (31-48). Washington, D.C.: American Psychological Association. Retrieved from http://proxy1.ncu.edu/login?url=http://search.ebscohost.com/login.aspx?direct=true&db=pzh&AN=2003-04376-003&site=ehost-live

McGuire, M.T., Wing, R.R., Klem, M.L., Lang, W., & Hills, J.O. (1999). What predicts weight regain in a group of successful weight losers? *Journal of Consulting and Clinical Psychology, 67*(2), 177-185.

McIver, S., McGartland, M., & O'Halloran, P. "Overeating is not about the food": Women describe their experience of a yoga treatment program for binge eating. *Qualitative Health Research, 19*, 1234-1245.

Medical insurance: Obesity, a rampant silent killer. (2006, February). *Life Insurance International.* Retrieved from http://proquest.umi.com.proxy1.ncu.edu/pqdweb?did=984684291&sid=2&Fmt=3 &clientld=52110&RQT=309&VName=PQD

Mela, D.J. (2006). Eating for pleasure or just wanting to eat? Reconsidering sensory hedonic responses as a driver of obesity. *Appetite, 47,* 10-17.

Millward, D.J. (1998). Metabolic demands for amino acids and the human dietary requirement. *Journal of Nutrition,* 2563S-2576S.

Morrill, A.C., & Chinn, C.D. (2004). The obesity epidemic in the United States. *Journal of Public Health Policy, 25(¾),* 353-367.

Morris, K., et al. (1999). Glycemic index, cardiovascular disease, and obesity. *Nutrition Reviews, 57,* 273-276.

Murray, M.T., & Beutler, J. (1996). *Understanding fats and oils.* Encinitas, CA: Progressive Health Publishing.

Mussell, M.P., Mitchell, J.E., Weller, C.L., Raymond, N.C., Crow, S.J., & Crosby, R.D. (1995). Onset of binge eating, dieting, obesity, and mood disorders among subjects seeking treatment for binge eating disorder. *International Journal of Eating Disorders, 17(4),* 395-401.

National Weight Control Registry. Retrieved April 8, 2011 from http://www.nwcr.ws/

Nelson, J.K., et al. (1994). *Mayo Clinic diet manual: A handbook of nutrition practices* (7th ed.). St. Louis, MO: Mosby.

Neumark-Sztainer, D. & Haines, J. (2004). Psychosocial and behavioral consequences of

obesity. In Thompson, K.J. (Ed.), *Handbook of eating disorders and obesity* (pp. 349-371). Hoboken, NJ: John Wiley & Sons.

Netzer, C.T. (2003). *The complete book of food counts.* New York, NY: Dell Publishing.

Nicholl, C.G., Polak, J.M., & Bloom, S.R. (1985). The hormonal regulation of food intake, digestion, and absorption. *Annual Review of Nutrition, 5,* 213-239.

Nijs, I.M.T., Muris, P., Euser, A.S., & Franken, I.H.A. (2010). Differences in attention to food and food intake between overweight/obese and normal weight subjects under conditions of hunger and satiety. *Appetite, 54,* 243-254.

Nobels, F., et al. (1989). Weight reduction with a high protein, low carbohydrate, caloric restricted diet: Effects on blood pressure, glucose, and insulin levels. *Netherlands Journal of Medicine, 35,* 295-302.

O'Brien, C. Does mindful eating help you eat less or just better? Matherways Life Institute on Aging. Retrieved from http://www.matherlifeways.com/documents/MLIA/MLWOrangePaper_MindfulEating_2.pdf

Ochsner, & Gross (2008). Cognitive emotional regulation: Insights from social cognitive and affective neuroscience. *Current Directions is Psychological Science, 17*(2), 153-158.

Olshansky, S.J., Passaro, D.J., Hershow, R.C., Layden, J., Carnes, B.A., Brody, J., ... Ludwig, D.S. (2005). A potential decline in life expectancy in the United States in the 21st century. *The New England Journal of Medicine, 352*(11), 1138-1146.

Palmeira, A.L., Teixeira, P.J., Branco, T.L., Martins, S.S., Minderico, C.S., Barata, J.T., ... Sardinha, L.B. (2007). Predicting short-term weight loss using four leading health behavior change theories. *International journal of Behavioral Nutrition and Physical Activity, 4*(14), 1-12. doi:10.1186/1479-5868-4-14

Palmer, B. (2000). *Helping people with eating disorders: A clinical guide to assessment and treatment.* West Sussex PO19 8SQ, England: John Wiley & Sons.

Papies, E.K., Stroebe, W., & Aarts, H. (2008). Healthy cognition: Processes of self-regulatory success in restrained eating. *Personality and Social Psychology Bulletin, 34*, 1290-1300.

Persaud, N. (2010). Interviewing. In N. Salkind (Ed.), *Encyclopedia of research design.* (pp. 633-637). Thousand Oaks, CA: SAGE Publications, Inc. doi: 10.4135/9781412961288.n197

Peterson, C.E., Wonderlich, S.A., Mitchell, J.E., & Crow, S.J. (2004). Integrative cognitive therapy for bulimia nervosa. In K.J. Thompson (Ed.), *Handbook of eating disorders and obesity* (pp. 245-262). Hoboken, NJ: John Wiley & Sons.

Petty, N.J., Thomson, O.P., & Stew, G. (2012). Ready for a paradigm shift: Part 2: Introducing qualitative research methodologies and methods. *Manual Therapy, 17*, 378-384.

Phelan, S., & Wadden, T.A. (2004). Behavioral assessment of obesity. In K.J. Thompson (Ed.), *Handbook of eating disorders and obesity* (pp. 393-420). Hoboken, NJ: John Wiley & Sons.

Pieke, B., et al. (2000). Treatment of hypertriglyceridemia by two diets rich either in unsaturated fatty acids or in carbohydrates: Effects on lipoprotein subclasses, lipolytic enzymes, lipid transfer proteins, insulin, and leptin. *International Journal of Obesity, 24*, 1286-1296.

Pike, K., Devlin, M.J., & Loeb, K. L. (2004). Cognitive behavioral therapy in the treatment of anorexia nervosa, bulimia nervosa, and binge eating disorder. In K.J. Thompson (Ed.), *Handbook of eating disorders and obesity* (pp. 130-162). Hoboken, NJ: John Wiley & Sons.

Pilkis, S.J., et al. (1988). Hormonal regulation of hepatic gluconeogenesis and glycolysis. *Annual Review of Biochemistry, 57*, 755-783.

Piran, N. (2005). Prevention of eating disorders: A review of outcome evaluation research. *Israeli Journal of Psychiatry and Related Sciences, (42)3*, pp. 172-177.

Polit, D.F., & Beck, C.T. (2004). *Nursing research, principles, and methods.* Philadelphia, PA: Lippincott, Williams, & Wilkins.

Ponterotto, J. (2005). Qualitative research in counseling psychology: a primer on research paradigms and philosophy of science. *Journal of Counseling Psychology, 52* (2), 126–136. Retrieved from http://proxy1.ncu.edu/login?url=http://search.ebscohost.com/login.aspx?direct=true&db=bth&AN=16753639&site=ehost-live

Porter, S. (2007). Validity, trustworthiness and rigour: Reasserting realism in qualitative research. *Journal of Advanced Nursing, 60*(1), 79-86.

Powell, L., Calvin, J., & Calvin, J. (2007). Effective obesity treatments. *American Psychologist, 62*(3), 234-246. doi:10.1037/0003-066X.62.3.234

Power, M.L., & Schulkin, J. (2009). The Evolution of Obesity. Baltimore, MD: The Johns Hopkins Press.

Presnell, K., Pells, J., Stout, A., & Musante, G. (2008). Sex differences in the relation of weight loss self-efficacy, binge eating, and depressive symptoms to weight loss success in a residential obesity treatment program. *Eating Behaviors, 9*, 170-180.

Rabast, U., Schonborn, J., & Kasper, H. (1979). Dietetic treatment of obesity with low- and high-carbohydrate diets: Comparative studies and clinical results. *International Journal of Obesity, 3*(3), 201-211.

Reed, W.D., et al. (1984). The effects of insulin and glucagon on ketone-body turnover. *Biochemistry, 221*, 439-444.

Reeds, P.J., & Hutchens, T.W. (1994). Protein requirements: From nitrogen balance to functional impact. *Journal of Nutrition*, 1754S-1963-S.

Reville, W. (2006, January 12). Being a little overweight should not exercise us too much. *Irish Times*, p. 15. Retrieved from http://proquest.umi.com.proxy1.ncu.edu/pqdweb?did=967036751&sid=4&Fmt=3&clientld=52110&RQT=309&VName=PQD

Richter, E.A., Ploug, T., & Galbo, H. (1985). Increased muscle glucose uptake after exercise. *Diabetes, 34*, 1041-1048.

Rieger, E. (2009). The use of motivational enhancement strategies for the maintenance of weight

loss among obese individuals: a preliminary investigation. *Diabetes, Obesity and Metabolism, 11*, 637-640. doi:10.1111/j.1463-1326.2008.01027.x

Robinson, A.L., Kosmerly, S., Mansfield-Green, S., & LaFrance, G. (2013). Disordered eating behavior in an undergraduate sample: Associations among gender, body mass index, and difficulties in emotion regulation. *Canadian Journal of Behavioral Science, 1-7*. doi: 10.1037/a0031123

Ruiz, S.Y., Pepper, A., & Wilfley, D.E. (2004). Obesity and body image among ethnically diverse children and adolescents. In Thompson, K.J. (Ed.), *Handbook of eating disorders and obesity* (pp. 656-678). Hoboken, NJ: John Wiley & Sons.

Ryan, R.M., Bernstein, J.H., & Brown, K.W. (2010). Weekends, work, and well-being: Psychological need satisfactions and day of the week effects on mood, vitality, and physical symptoms. *Journal of Social and Clinical Psychology, 29*, 95-122.

Sassaroli, S., & Ruggiero, G.M. (2005). The role of stress in the association between low self-esteem, perfectionism, and worry, and eating disorders. *International Journal of Eating Disorders, 37*, 135-141.

Schlosser, E. (2001). *Fast food nation: The dark side of the all American meal.* New York, NY: Houghton Mifflin Company.

Scriver, C.R., et al. (1985). Normal plasma amino acid values in adults: The influence of some common physiological variables. *Metabolism, 34*, 868-873.

Schmeichel, B.J., & Baumeister, R.F. (2004). Self regulatory strength. In Roy F. Baumeister & Kathleen D. Vohs (Eds.), *handbook of self regulation: Research, theory, and applications* (84-98). New York, NY: The Guildford Press,

Sears, B., & Lawren, B. (1995). *Enter the zone.* New York, NY: Harper Collins.

Segar, M.L., Updegraff, J.A., Zikmund-Fisher, B.J., & Richardson, C.R. (2012). Physical activity advertisements that feature daily well-being improve autonomy and body image in overweight women but not men. *Journal of Obesity, 2012*(354721), 1-19. doi:10.1155/201 54721

Sheldon, K.M., & Elliott, A.J. (1998). Not all personal goals are personal: Comparing autonomous and controlled reasons as predictors of effort and attainment. *Personality and Social Psychology Bulletin, 24*, 546-557.

Sims, E.A. (1974). Studies in human hyperphagia. *Treatment and management of obesity.* New York, NY: Harper and Row.

Slochower, J., & Kaplan, S.P. (1980). Anxiety, perceived control, and eating in obese and normal weight persons. *Appetite, 1*, 75-83.

Smolak, L., & Murnen, S.K. (2004). A feminist approach to eating disorders. In Thompson, K.J. (Ed.), *Handbook of eating disorders and obesity* (pp. 590-605). Hoboken, NJ: John Wiley & Sons.

Smolak, L., & Striegel-Moore, R.H. (2004). Future directions in eating disorder and obesity research. In K.J. Thompson (Ed.), *Handbook of eating disorders and obesity* (pp. 738-753). Hoboken, NJ: John Wiley & Sons.

Souba, W.W., Smith, R.J., & Wilmore, D.W. (1985). Glutamine metabolism by the intestinal tract. *Journal of Parenteral Enteral Nutrition, 9*, 608-617.

Stewart, K.J., Bacher, A.C., Turner, K., et al. (2005). Exercise and risk factors associated with metabolic syndrome in older adults. *American Journal of Preventative Medicine, 28*(1), 9-18.

Stice, E., & Hoffman, E. (2004). Eating disorder prevention programs. In K.J. Thompson (Ed.), *Handbook of eating disorders and obesity* (pp. 33-57). Hoboken, NJ: John Wiley & Sons.

Stordy, B.J., et al. (1977). Weight gain, thermic effects of glucose and resting metabolic rate during recovery from anorexia nervosa. *American Journal of Clinical Nutrition, 30*, 138.

Swinburn, B.A., et al. (2011). The global obesity pandemic: Shaped by global drives and local environments. *Lancet, 378*(9793), 804-814.

Tantleff-Dunn-Dunn, S., Gokle-LaRose, J., & Peterson, R.D. (2004). Interpersonal psychotherapy for the treatment of anorexia nervosa, bulimia nervosa, and binge eating disorder. In K.J. Thompson (Ed.), *Handbook of eating disorders and obesity* (pp. 163-185). Hoboken, NJ: John Wiley & Sons.

Teixeira, P.J., Silva, M.N., Coutinho, S.R., Palmeira, A.L., Mata, J., Vieira, P.N., . . . Sardinha, L.B. (2010). Mediators of weight loss and weight loss maintenance in middle-aged women. *Obesity, 18*, 725-735. doi:10.1038/oby.2009.281

Thaler, J.P., et al. (2012). Obesity is associated with hypothalamic injury in rodents and humans. *The Journal of Clinical Investigation, 122*(1).

Thompson, J.K. (Ed.). (2004). *Handbook of eating disorders and obesity.* Hoboken, NJ: John Wiley & Sons.

Thompson, K.M., & Wonderlich, S.A. (2004). Childhood sexual abuse and eating disorders. In Thompson, K.J. (Ed.), *Handbook of eating disorders and obesity* (pp. 679-694). Hoboken, NJ: John Wiley & Sons.

Thorne, A., & Wahren, J. (1989). Diet-induced thermogenesis in well-trained subjects. *Clinical Physiology*, 295-305.

Tice, D.M., Bratslavsky, E., & Baumeister, R.F. (2001). Emotional distress regulation takes precedence over impulse control: If you feel bad, do it! *Journal of Personality and Social Psychology, 80*(1), 53-67. doi:10.1037//0022-3514.80.1.53

Traxinger, R.R., & Marshall, S. (1989). Role of amino acids in modulating glucose-induced desensitization of the glucose transport system. *Journal of Biological Chemistry, 264*, 20910-20916.

Tuckett, A.G. (2005). Part II. Rigour in qualitative research: Complexities and solutions. *Nurse Researcher, 13*(1), 29-42.

Underwood, A, & Adler, J. (Jan. 17, 2005). Diet and genes. *Newsweek, 40*, 8.

van den Bos, R., Harteveld, M., & Stoop, H. (2009). Stress and decision-making in humans: Performance is related to cortisol reactivity, albeit differently in men and women. *Psychoneuroendocrinology, 34*, 1449-1458. doi:10.1016/j.psyneuen.2009.04.016

van den Bos, R., Homberg, R., & de Visser, L., (2013). A critical review of sex differences in decision-making tasks: Focus on the Iowa Gambling Task. *Behavioural Brain Research, 1*(238), 95-108. doi:10.1016/j.bbr.2012.10.002

Verplanken, B., Walker, L., Davis, A., & Jurasek, M. (2008). Context change and travel mode choice: Combining the habit discontinuity and self-activation hypotheses. *Journal of Environmental Psychology, 28*, 121-127.

Verstuyf, J., Vansteenkiste, M., Soenens, B., & Boone, L. (2013). Daily ups and downs in women's binge eating symptoms: The role of basic psychological needs, general self-control, and emotional eating. *Journal of Social and Clinical Psychology, 32*(3), 335-361.

Vohs, K.D., & Heatherton, T.F. (2000). Self-regulatory failure: A resource-depletion approach. *Psychological Science, 11*, 249-254.

Wang, et al., (2009). Evidence of gender differences in the ability to inhibit brain activation elicited by food stimulation. *Proceedings of the National Academy of Sciences, 106*(4), 1249-1254.

Wardle, J. (1988). Cognitive control of eating. *Journal of Psychosomatic Research, 32*(6), 607-612.

Weinberg, A., & Klonsky, E. D. (2009). Measurement of emotion dysregulation in adolescents. *Psychological Assessment, 21*, 616–621. doi:10.1037/a0016669

Weinstein, A.R., Sesso, H.P., Lee, I.M., et al. (2004). Relationship of physical activity versus body mass index with type II diabetes in women. *Journal of the American Medical Association, 292*, 10, 1188-9.

Weller, R.E., Cook, E.W., Avsar, K.B., & Cox, J.E. (2008). Obese women show greater delay discounting than healthy-weight women. *Appetite, 51*, 563-569.

Werrij, M.Q., Jansen, A., Mulkens, S., Elgersma, H.J., Ament, A.J.H.A., & Hospers, H.J. (2009). Adding cognitive therapy to dietetic treatment is associated with less relapse in obesity. *Journal of Psychosomatic Research, 67*, 315-324.

Wertheim, E.H., Paxton, S.J., & Blaney, S. (2004). Risk factors for the development of body image disturbances. In Thompson, K.J. (Ed.), *Handbook of eating disorders and obesity* (pp. 463-494). Hoboken, NJ: John Wiley & Sons.

Wessel, T.R., Arant, C.B., Olson, M.B., et al. (2004). Relationship of physical fitness versus body mass index with coronary artery disease and cardiovascular events in women. *Journal of the American Medical Association, 292*(10), 1179-87.

Westphal, S.A., Gannon, M.C., & Nutrall, F.Q. (1990). Metabolic response to glucose ingested with various amounts of protein. *American Journal of Clinical Nutrition, 62*, 267-272.

Whitney, E.N., & Rolfes, S.R. (1996). *Understanding nutrition,* (7th ed.). St. Paul, MN: West Publishing Company.

Willett, W.C., Manson, J.E., Stampfer, M.J., Colditz, G.A., Rosner, B.R., Speizer, F.E., & Hennekens, C.H. (1995). Weight, weight change, and coronary heart disease in women: Risk within 'normal' weight range. *Journal of the American Medical Association, 273*, 461-465.

Williams, P., Surwit, R., Babyak, M., & McCaskill, C. (1998). Personality predictors of mood related to dieting. *Journal of Consulting and Clinical Psychology, 66*(6), 994-1004. doi:10.1037/0022-006X.66.6.994

Willig, C. (2008). Introducing qualitative research in psychology: Adventures in theory and method (2nd ed.). Maidenhead, England: McGraw Hill/Open University Press. Retrieved from http://site.ebrary.com.proxy1.ncu.edu/lib/ncent/docDetail.action?docID=10246330 ISBN: 9780335236343

Wilson, T. (1999). Eating disorders and addictions. *Drugs and Society, (15)*½, 87-101.

Wing, R.R., Fava, J.L., Phelan, S., McCaffery, J., Papandonatos, G., Gorin, A.A., & Tate, D.F. (2008). Maintaining large weight losses: The role of behavioral and psychological factors. *Journal of Consulting and Clinical Psychology, 76*(6), 1015-1021. doi: 10.1037/a0014159

Wolfe, B.M. (1995). Potential role of raising dietary protein intake for reducing risk of atherosclerosis. *Canadian Journal of Cardiology, 11*, 127G-131G.

Woods, S.C., et al. (1998). Signals that regulate food intake and energy homeostasis. *Science, 280*, 1378-1383.

Woolhouse, H., Knowles, A., & Crafti, N. (2013). Adding mindfulness to CBT programs for binge eating: A mixed-methods evaluation. *Eating Disorders: The Journal of Treatment & Prevention, 20*(4), 321-339. doi:10.1080/10640266.2012.691791

Yamada, T., et al. (1995). *Textbook of gastroenterology, (2nd ed.).* Philadelphia, PA: J.B. Lippincott Company.

Young, D.B., et al. (1984). Effects of sodium intake on steady-state potassium excretion. *American Journal of Physiology, 246*, F772-F778.

Young, V.R., & Marchini, J.S. (1990). Mechanisms and nutritional significance of metabolic responses to altered intakes of protein and amino acids, with reference to nutritional adaption in humans. *American Journal of Clinical Nutrition, 51*, 270-289.

Zheng, H., Lenard, N., Shin, A., & Berthoud, H. (2009, June). Appetite control and energy balance regulation in the modern world: Reward-driven brain overrides repletion signals. International Journal of Obesity, *33*(Suppl 2), S8-S13.

Zlomke, K.R., & Hahn, K.S. (2010). Cognitive emotion regulation strategies: Gender differences and associations to worry. *Personality and Individual Differences, 48*, 408-413.

Zoladz, P.R., Warnecke, A.J., Woelke, S.A., Burke, H.M., Frigo, R.M., Pisansky, J.M., . . . Talbot, J.N. (2013). Pre-learning stress that is temporally removed from acquisition exerts sex-specific effects on long-term memory. *Neurobiology of Learning and Memory, 100*, 77-87.

ABOUT THE AUTHORS

Joe Klemczewski, PhD, has multiple degrees in physical and health sciences, including a doctorate in health education. He is the founder of The Diet Doc, LLC (thedietdoc.com), *ALPHA Mag: The Evolution of Fitness* (alphamagonline.com), and The Shadow Foundation (inspire-themovement.org). He has contributed to top magazines as a science editor, feature writer, and columnist for two decades, Dr. Joe maintains his *Diet Doc* newspaper column and is the co-author of *The Diet Docs' Guide to Permanent Weight Loss: Secrets to Metabolic Transformation* (Harvest House Publishers 2008) and the author of *Metabolic Transformation: The Ultimate Fat-Loss Guide* (iUniverse 2003).

Kori Propst, PhD(c), earned a bachelor's degree in exercise physiology, a master's degree in community counseling, and is in the dissertation process of her doctorate in health psychology and behavioral medicine. She has contributed to magazines around the world and is a popular blogger and workshop facilitator. Kori created *The Mental Edge Program* to help clients reach their fullest potential with health and performance goals by equipping them with life skill and mindset training tools. She is the Wellness Director of The Diet Doc, LLC, and manages the licensing operation program for Diet Doc clinicians with dozens of locations in the United States, Canada, Great Britain, and Australia.